BLOOD PRESSURE

MONITORING JOURNAL

BLOOD PRESSURE MONITORING JOURNAL

A Hypertension Diary and Log

Milton D. Lee, M.S.
and
Joyce E. Lee, M.S

Library of Congress Control Number:		2010917435
ISBN:	Hardcover	978-1-4568-2173-9
	Softcover	978-1-4568-2172-2
	Ebook	978-1-4568-2174-6

The content in this book is provided for general informational purposes only and is not meant to substitute for the advice provided by a medical professional. This information is not intended to diagnose or treat any medical problems or substitute for appropriate medical care. If you have or suspect that you have a medical problem, promptly contact your health care provider. Never disregard professional medical advice or delay in seeking it because of something you have read in this book. If you utilize any information provided in this book, you do so at your own risk and you specifically waive any right to make any claim against the author and publisher, its officers, directors, employees or representatives as the result of the use of such information.

** See a doctor promptly if you: have more than one daily reading of 140/90 or higher, have frequent headaches, especially in the morning, feel short of breath and lack stamina, feel dizzy, develop a chronic red face, have frequent nose bleeds and/or have fainting spells.**

This book was printed in the United States of America.

To order additional copies of this book, contact:
Xlibris Corporation
1-888-795-4274
www.Xlibris.com
Orders@Xlibris.com
90623

CONTENTS

Part One—Introduction

Part Two—Recordation and monitoring

"A merry heart does good like a medicine"
Proverbs 17:22

Blood Pressure
Monitoring Journal
A Hypertension Diary and Log
by Milton D. Lee and Joyce E. Lee

"A simplistic way to monitor
Blood Pressure"

This Journal belongs to

_____

From_____ To_____

DEDICATION

This journal is dedicated to all those who
are experiencing symptoms of High Blood Pressure.
Our prayer is by monitoring your Blood Pressure you
will take an active role over managing your symptoms
in addition, get the necessary help from your health care professional.

INTRODUCTION

How to use the journal?

The purpose and design of this Blood Pressure Monitoring Journal is to help keep track of your blood pressure reading. It is designed so that the recording of your blood pressure can be done easily any time of the day or night. This journal is simplistic and not complicated in design; therefore, the blood pressure reading you take and record are easily understood. All the pages have designed areas for recordation of the systolic reading, and diastolic reading, day of the week, date, pulse rate, and time of day. Utilize the nutritional and activity logs to input your food intake and exercises during that day or within the week. It also has a notes and questions section for any thoughts that might come to mine that you may want to ask your doctor.

Why keep a blood pressure journal?

One simple personal action of self-monitoring your blood pressure reading and recording them is an effective way of reducing hypertension. There have been some cases where it has lead to eliminating the need for medication. As with other activities, when it is written down (documented, organized, monitored) it is easier for you to point to and have available for review with your doctor. It gives him or her an accurate view of how your blood pressure is on a daily bases. You can further chart any change in your blood pressure, whether dramatic or slight, over a period of time. Therefore, by maintaining your own blood pressure reading via log and journal puts you in charge of your own regimen. In addition to keeping a log on your blood pressure, you can chart what foods you eat, activities that you do (walking, jogging, swimming, yoga) during the day. You can further write down thoughts that might come to mind that maybe questions to ask your personal health care provider or physician on your next appointment.

Tracking Blood Pressure

Before we start to track your blood pressure, let us define blood pressure. Some people may think our blood flows through our arteries in a steady stream like water through a faucet. However, this is not true. Rather it courses through the body in pulses produced by each contraction of the heart. Therefore, the result is blood pressure. Blood Pressure is the force your arteries use to push blood through the arteries and venous system. This process is analogous to a water hose. Therefore, if the water hose is larger than the amount of water flowing through it water does not back up. However, it the hose is smaller than the force of water attempting to go through, the water cannot move through freely, and begins to build back up. In regards to the human heart, when vascular resistance increases, the heart must work harder to overcome this resistance. As a result, the blood backs up much like the water in the narrow hose, and this causes hypertension.

In 1988, a report from the Joint National Committee on Detection, Evaluation, and Treatment of High Blood Pressure came out to establish exactly what level of high blood pressure is too high. The numbers reported that blood pressure above or equal to 140/90 is considered high. This revelation came after years of research to discover at what blood pressure the body begins to exhibit adverse effects. The measurement always includes two numbers that represent two basic phases, called the systolic and diastolic pressures. These are representing the high and low pressure of each beat. When we hear, the weather forecasters talk about the barometer of our weather, our blood pressure readings are expressed in the same units of measure: millimeters of mercury. Be aware that if your blood pressure is 139/89, this does not mean you are not at risk.

Having to track and check your blood pressure is painless and quick. It is usually preformed with the use of a stethoscope and a sphygmomanometer (sphygmo means "Pulse"), which consists of an inflatable arm cuff attached to a column of mercury and a gauge. The cuff is wrapped around the upper arm just above the elbow, is inflated with air to compress the brachial artery, the major artery in the arm, to a pressure that shuts off all of the blood flow through the artery. As the cuff deflates, the person taking the blood pressure reading listens through a stethoscope placed on the brachial artery for the first audible beat (the sound of blood rushing back into the compressed artery) and notes the number on the gauge.

Prior to taking a reading of your blood pressure, relax in a quiet room, seated in a chair or recline on a sofa for approximately five minutes and at least thirty minutes after consuming caffeine or smoking. Take multiple readings, at least two; wait approximately two to three minutes between the readings, one taken in each arm. Do not talk during the reading. It is important to make sure you have the right-size blood pressure cuff in order to get an accurate blood pressure reading. If the cuff is too small for a large arm, the pressure reading may be elevated above the true value because the cuff has to squeeze harder to compress the artery. It is less common for the reading to be low if the cuff is too large.

It is extremely important to make sure your blood pressure reading is as accurate as possible. One-way to ensure you get a proper reading is to keep your arm at heart level. Therefore, make sure your arm is elevated to your heart level. This position should give the most precise and accurate reading.

There are newer technologies in monitoring, such as wrist and finger cuffs with digital readouts, and the modernization of the stethoscope and sphygmomanometer to one unit cuff and the other unit issues a read out. The newer technology of Blood Pressure readout monitors, whether wrist, finger cuffs or inflatable arm cuff combination with readout monitor are now available for a nominal price in several pharmacies and drug stores. Whatever type of device you choose, have your doctor inspect it for accurate readings that you have the correct cuff size and to make sure you are using it properly. Self-monitoring, though a credible means of keeping track of your blood pressure, it is advisable for you to do so in conjunction with your physician's professional monitoring and guidance.

How Blood Pressure works.

Every time your heart beats, the walls of your arteries stretch, between beats, the arteries relax. A blood pressure (BP) reading reflects the force of blood against artery walls at these two times.

Systolic Blood Pressure:

The pressure generated by the heart immediately after it contracts or beats and represents the top number of the blood pressure reading. In this phase, the heart squeezes and pumps the blood into the arteries.

Diastolic Blood Pressure:

The number at which the last beat is audible. It is the arterial pressure maintained between heartbeats, when the heart is at rest. In this phase, the heart relaxes and fills with blood.

The combined ratio of systolic over diastolic reveals the relative pressure generated by the heart as it alternately pumps blood through the arteries and rests. Therefore, a blood pressure reading of 120/80 mm Hg represents a systolic pressure of 120 and a diastolic pressure of 80 mm Hg.

What the Numbers Mean

A blood pressure reading will indicate one of three states:

Hypotension	(Low Blood Pressure)
Normotension	(Normal Blood Pressure)
Hypertension	(High Blood Pressure)

The ideal is, Normotension, of course.

Blood Pressure Classification

Classification	Systolic	Diastolic
Optimal	under120	under 80
Normal	" 130	" 85
High Normal	130-139	85-89
Stage 1 Hypertension (mild)	140-159	90-99
Stage 2 Hypertension (moderate)	160-179	100-109
Stage 3 Hypertension (severe)	180+	110+

Times when Blood Pressure Alters

One should be aware of the fact that your blood pressure changes constantly throughout the day, depending on your activities, diet, environment, emotions, medications, and other factors. Blood normally is about 20 percent to 30 percent higher in waking hours than when you sleep, and higher in the afternoon than in the morning. Your highs might be missed depending on when you see the doctor and have your blood pressure taken. Some individuals have what is called "White Coat Hypertension". This is when the patient's blood pressure is higher than normal when it is being taken by a doctor or nurse in the process of an examination. When another person or the individual takes the pressure, the blood pressure would be in the normal range or lower. White Coat Hypertension highlights the inherent flaw of relying on one reading, or even several readings taken at about the same time.

A blood pressure reading normally follows a roller coaster path over the twenty-four-hour day. Blood pressure starts upwards before you habitually wake up, to prepare your body to function best in waking hours. Once you awaken, it surges or climbs abruptly through the morning and afternoon, peaks in late afternoon or early evening, and then slides to its trough in sleep. Example: Systolic BP ordinarily is about 25 to 30 mm Hg higher when you are awake than when you are asleep. Diastolic BP is about 15 to 20 mm Hg higher in the daytime.

Women and Blood Pressure Changes

A woman's menstrual cycle has an effect on her blood pressure. Her BP is a little higher in the week or so before the start of a menstrual period than it is in mid-month, at the time of ovulation. In women who use birth-control pills, both systolic / diastolic BP average about 4 to 5 mm Hg higher than in nonusers.

High Blood Pressure Risk Factors

Hypertension does not just happen. Numerous risk factors have been linked to the development of hypertension. These contributing factors includes diabetes, family history of hypertension, caffeine abuse, dangerous amounts of fatty molecules in the blood, excessive alcohol intake, race, gender, obesity, tobacco use, less than 30 grams of fiber in the diet, physical inactivity, stress, type A personality, and over consumption of animal fat and vegetable oil.

Within America and western culture, obesity has reached alarming proportions to where 30% of adults over the age of 20 are obese and over 60% of the population is overweight. Having excessive body fat can lead to, illnesses such as: type 2 diabetes, coronary artery disease, high blood pressure, stroke, high cholesterol, and triglycerides, sleep apnea, arthritis, and digestive problems. American researchers have found that the number leading cause of death in America is cardiovascular disease. Atherosclerosis, high blood pressure, high cholesterol, and high triglycerides are heart and blood vessel-related conditions that are directly linked to people's diet.

With these aforementioned risks in mind, change the way you view things, change the way you do things, and change your habits to include exercise, change your nutritional intake to include foods that change the biochemistry in your body, and begin to do things that will affect your health positively.

Hints to lower Blood Pressure

These changes may include the use only of organic milk products and goat's milk yogurt; avoid traditional mayonnaise made with soybean oil and switch to a canola-oil based mayonnaise. Avoid traditional cooking oils and use organic butter or coconut oil instead and artificial sweeteners that contain aspartame (NutraSweet) as it interferes with the blood sugar regulation in the body. Aspartame is also extremely toxic to the body because it is a neurotoxin (poisonous to the nervous system).

Add to the aforementioned, increase the consumption of plant foods in your diet. Some diets, such as vegetarian, typically contains less saturated fat and refined carbohydrates, and more potassium, complex carbohydrates, fiber, calcium, magnesium, vitamin C and essential fatty acids. In addition, double-blind studies have demonstrated that either fish oil supplements or flaxseed oil (both rich in omega-3 fatty acids) are very effective in lowering blood pressure.

Hints to lower Blood Pressure through Humor and Laughter

Scientific studies have shown that five to ten minutes of laughter first thing in the morning improves blood pressure levels. A mirthful laugher on a regular basis has a lower standing blood pressure than the average person does, however, when there is a good laugh initially the blood pressure increases, but then it decreases to levels below normal. While breathing then becomes deeper which sends oxygen enriched blood and nutrients throughout the body. Here is what according to research happens to you when you laugh:

- Your heart and lungs are stimulated.
- Your heart beats faster and your blood pressure rises temporarily
- You breathe deeper and oxygenate more blood
- Your body releases endorphins, your own natural painkillers, and you
- Your body produces more immune cells.
- You burn seventy-eight times as many calories as you would in a resting state.
- Your diaphragm, facial muscles, and internal organs all are moved around in what is sometimes, called "internal jogging."

After you have laughter, your muscles and arteries relax, also your blood pressure lowers and your pulse drops below normal.

Ten Principles to help manage your Blood Pressure

- ❖ **Prayer and Meditation**
- ❖ **Drink Water**
- ❖ **Eat Nutritiously**
- ❖ **Exercise Daily**
- ❖ **Breathe Deeply**
- ❖ **Listen to Soothing Music**
- ❖ **Practice Loving Self and Others**
- ❖ **Be Forgiving**
- ❖ **Gratitude**
- ❖ **Laughter and Humor**

References

Andrew, A. (2007), *Empowering your Health, Tennessee,* Thomas Nelson, Inc.

Moore, R. (2000), *The High Blood Pressure Solution: a scientifically proven program for preventing strokes and heart disease,* Vermont, Healing Arts Press

Smolensky, M. & Lamberg, L. (2000), *The Body clock guide to better health,* New York, Henry Holt and Company

Whitaker, J. (2000), *Reversing Hypertension: a vital new program to prevent, treat, and reduce high blood pressure,* New York, Warner Books

Some books that may be of interest for further information regarding high blood pressure are as follows:

Eat to beat High Blood Pressure by Robyn Webb, M.S., Jamy D. Ard, M.D., and Debra L. Gordon

Controlling High Blood Pressure the Natural Way by David L. Carroll and Wahida Karmally, M. S.

The amazing way to reverse Heart Disease Naturally by Eric R. Braverman, B.S., R.P.A.—C.

Empowering Your Health by Asa Andrew, M.D.

Laugh Yourself Healthy by Charles and Frances Hunter.

Drugs / Medications

Quantity	Description	Dosage

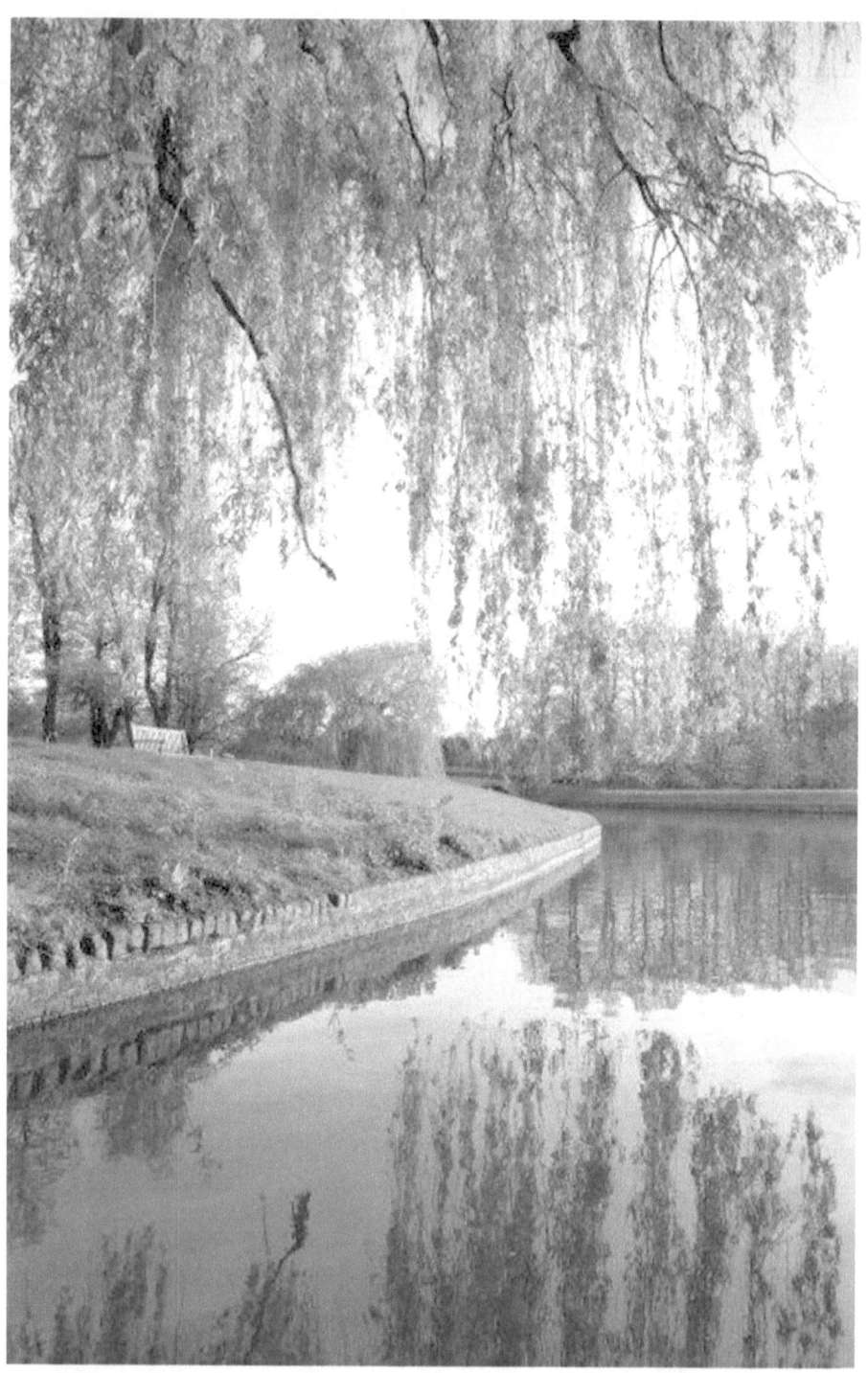

HYPERTENSION DIARY AND LOG

BLOOD PRESSURE LOG

Date / Day	Time	AM	PM	SYSTOLIC	DIASTOLIC	Pulse Rate

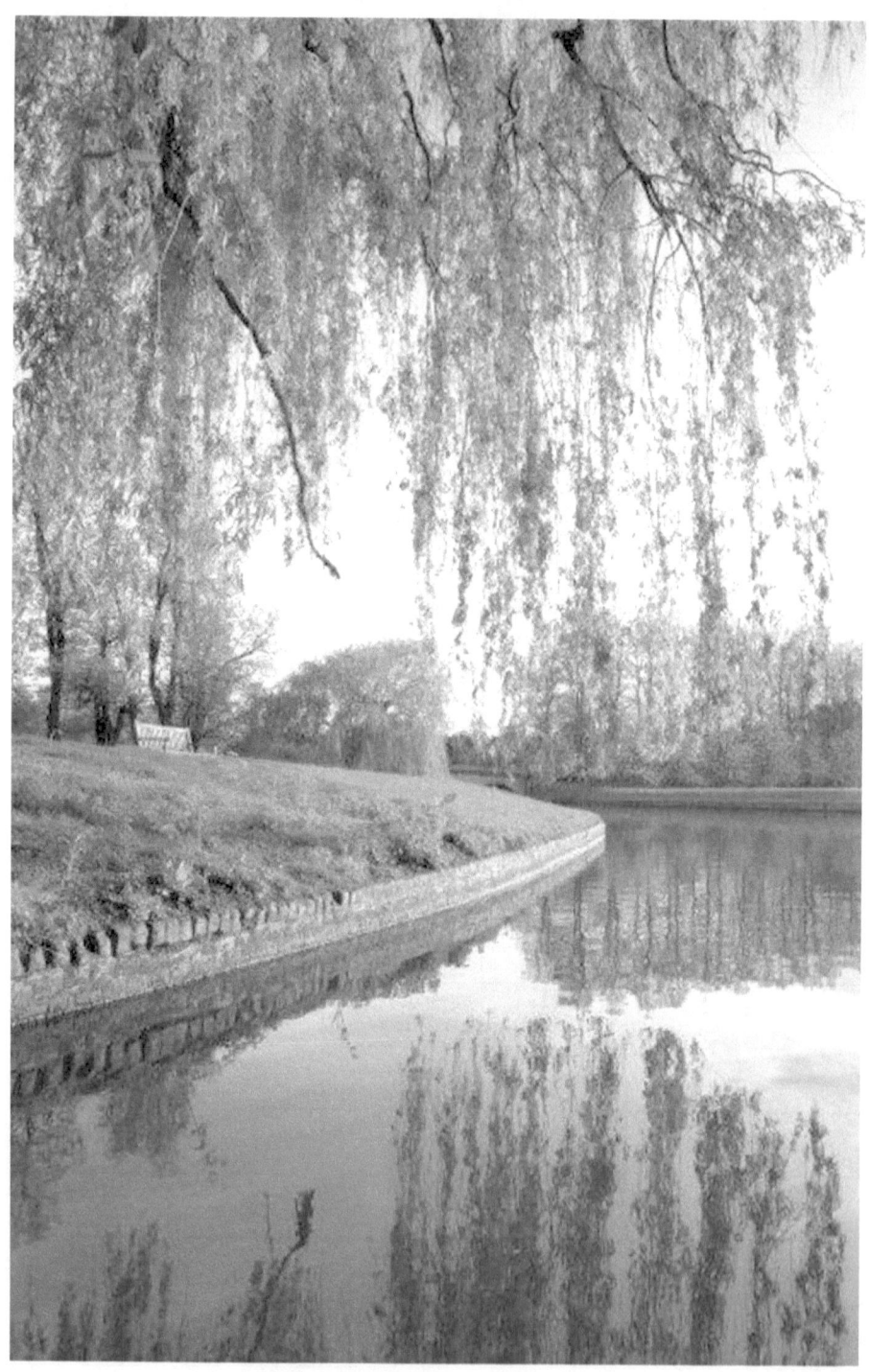

HYPERTENSION DIARY AND LOG

BLOOD PRESSURE LOG

Date / Day	Time	AM	PM	SYSTOLIC	DIASTOLIC	Pulse Rate

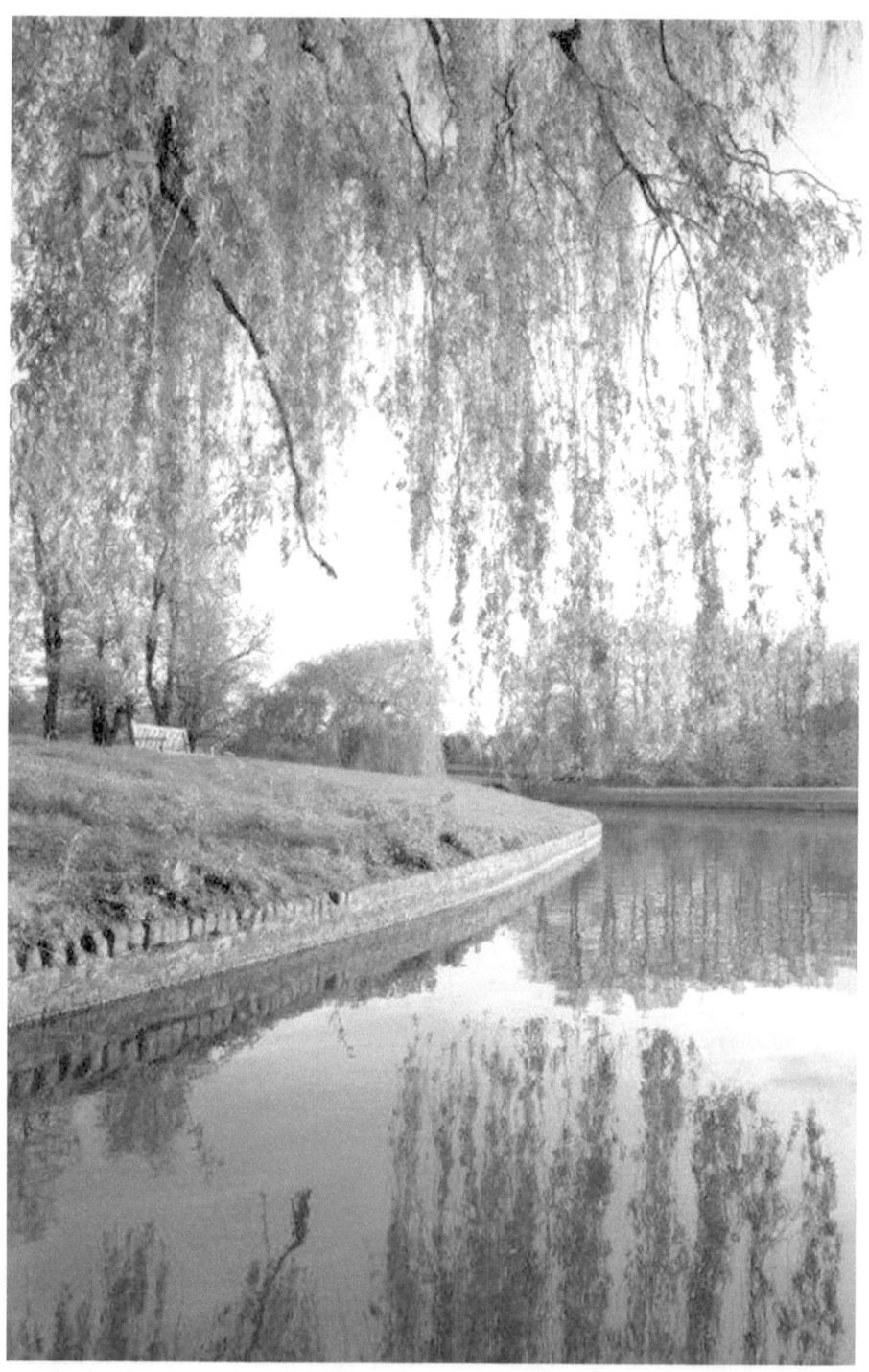

HYPERTENSION DIARY AND LOG

BLOOD PRESSURE LOG

Date / Day	Time	AM	PM	SYSTOLIC	DIASTOLIC	Pulse Rate

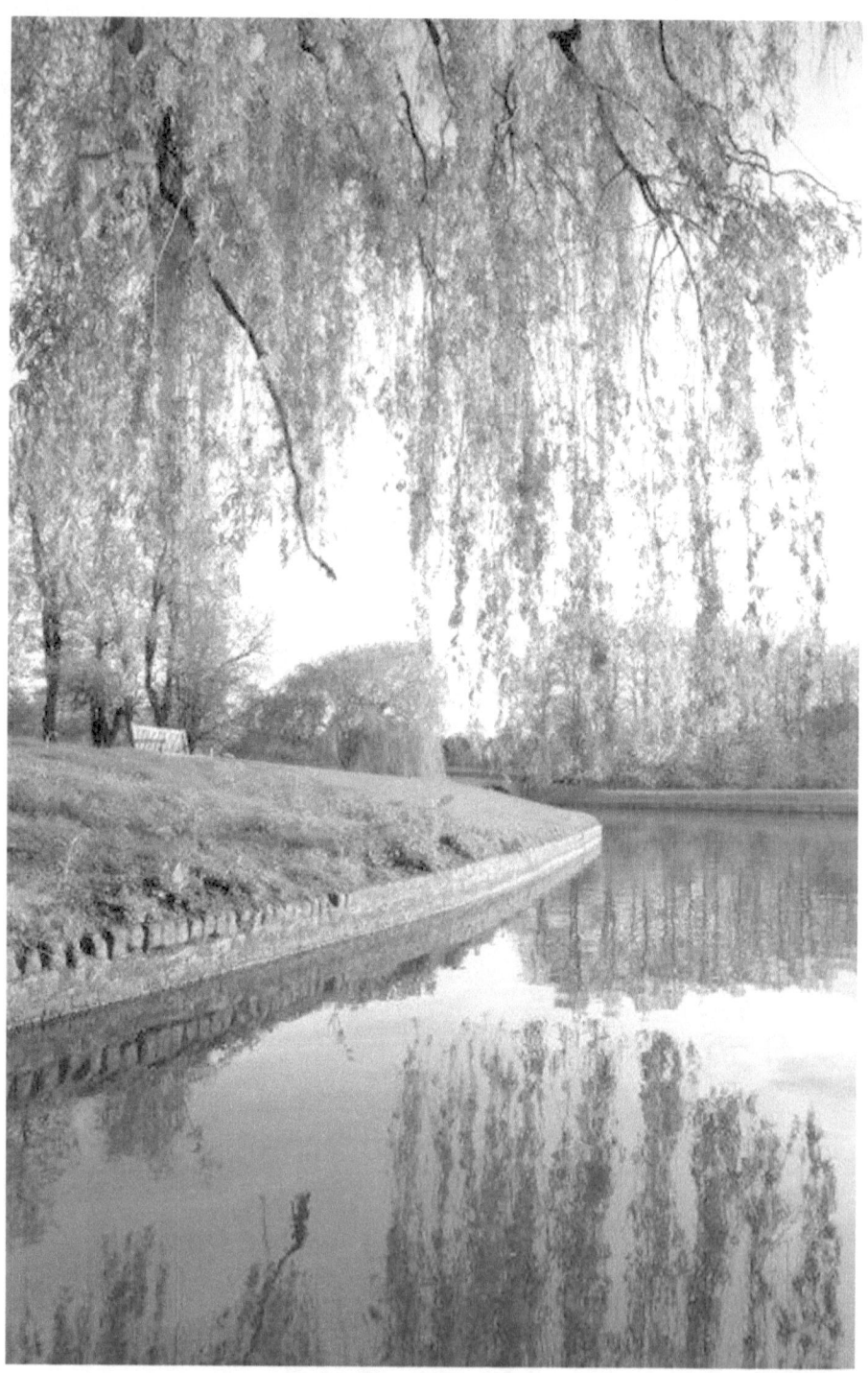

HYPERTENSION DIARY AND LOG

BLOOD PRESSURE LOG

Date / Day	Time	AM	PM	SYSTOLIC	DIASTOLIC	Pulse Rate

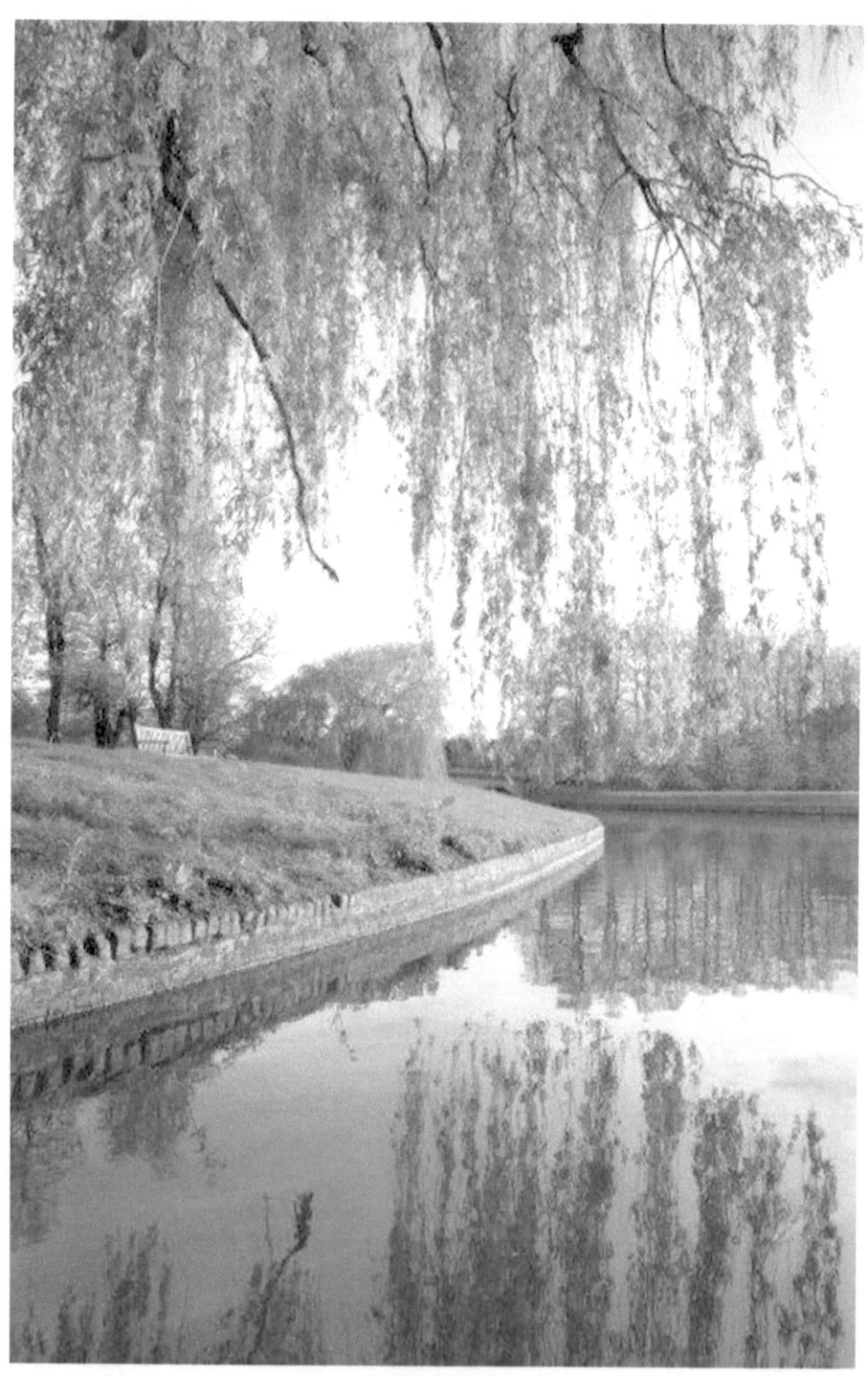

HYPERTENSION DIARY AND LOG

BLOOD PRESSURE LOG

Date / Day	Time	AM	PM	SYSTOLIC	DIASTOLIC	Pulse Rate

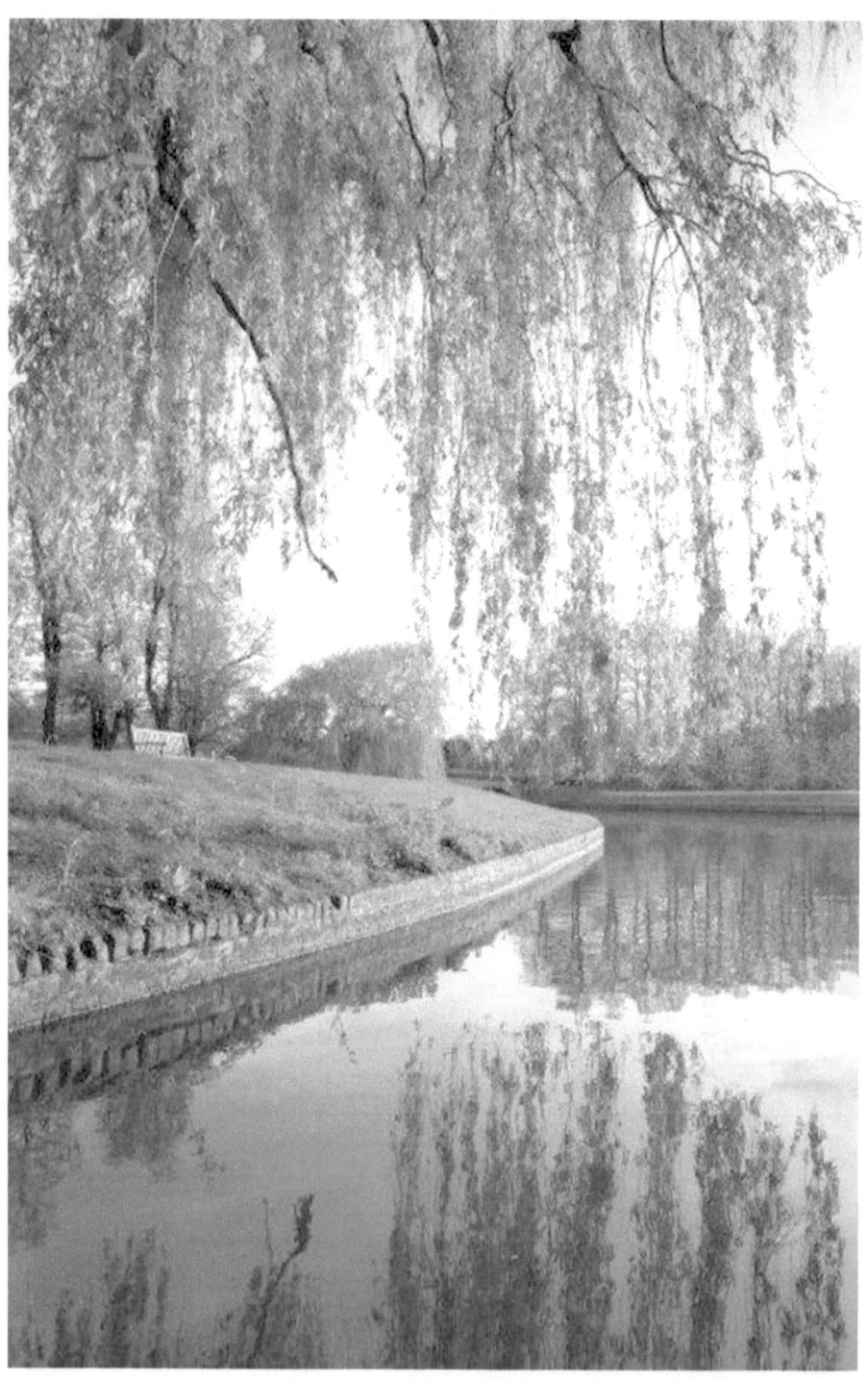

HYPERTENSION DIARY AND LOG

BLOOD PRESSURE LOG

Date / Day	Time	AM	PM	SYSTOLIC	DIASTOLIC	Pulse Rate

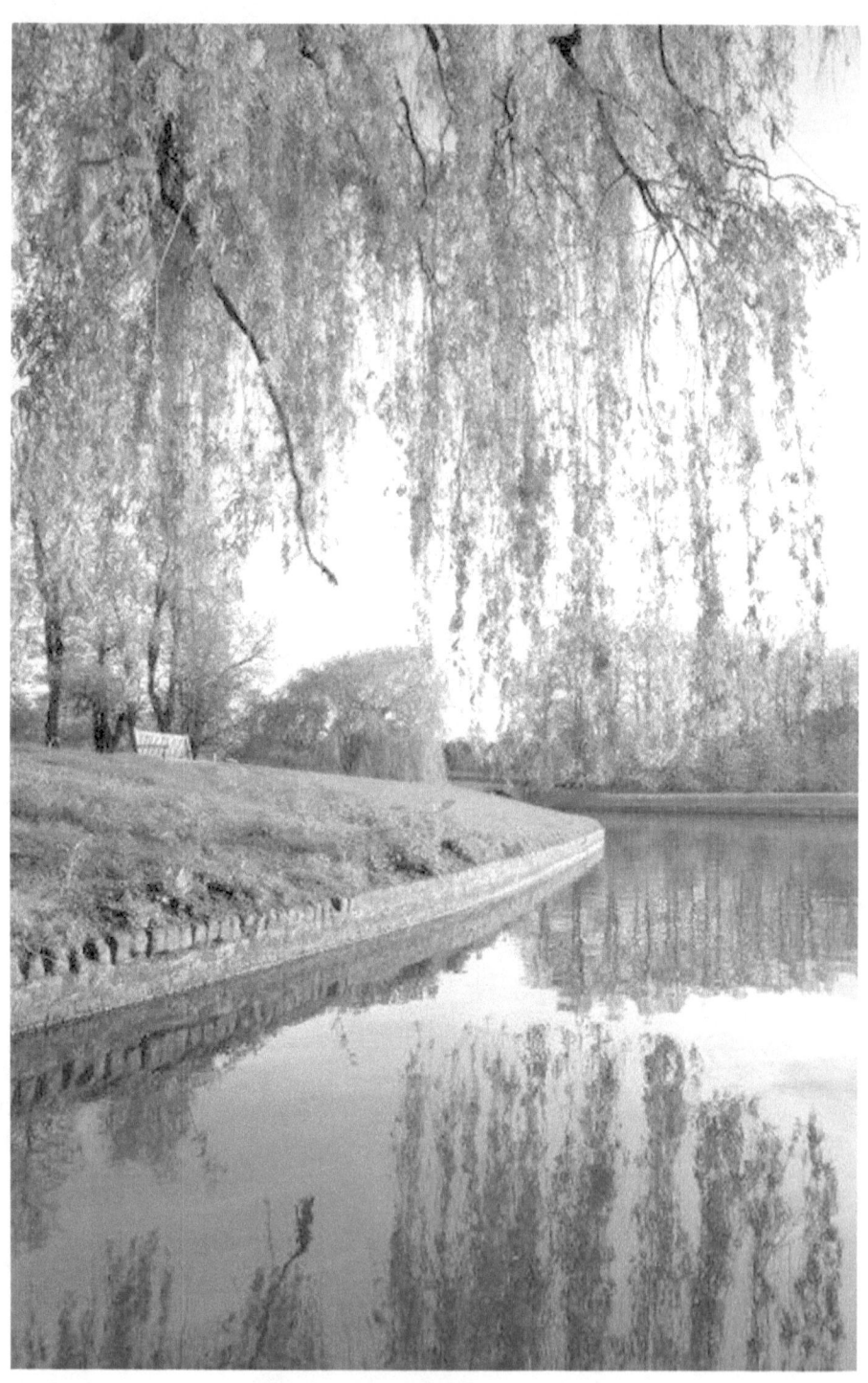

HYPERTENSION DIARY AND LOG

BLOOD PRESSURE LOG

Date / Day	Time	AM	PM	SYSTOLIC	DIASTOLIC	Pulse Rate

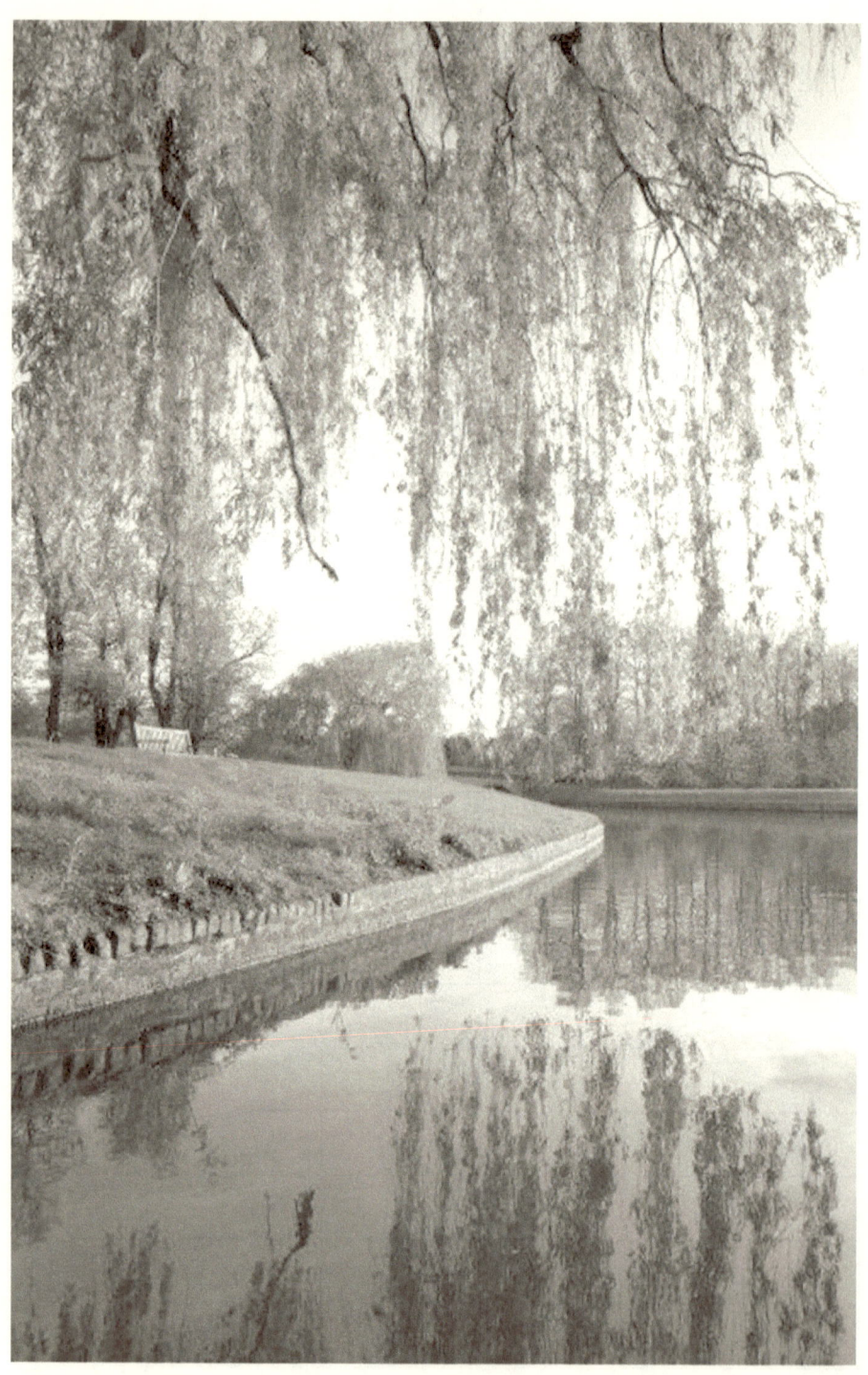

BLOOD PRESSURE LOG

Date / Day	Time	AM	PM	SYSTOLIC	DIASTOLIC	Pulse Rate

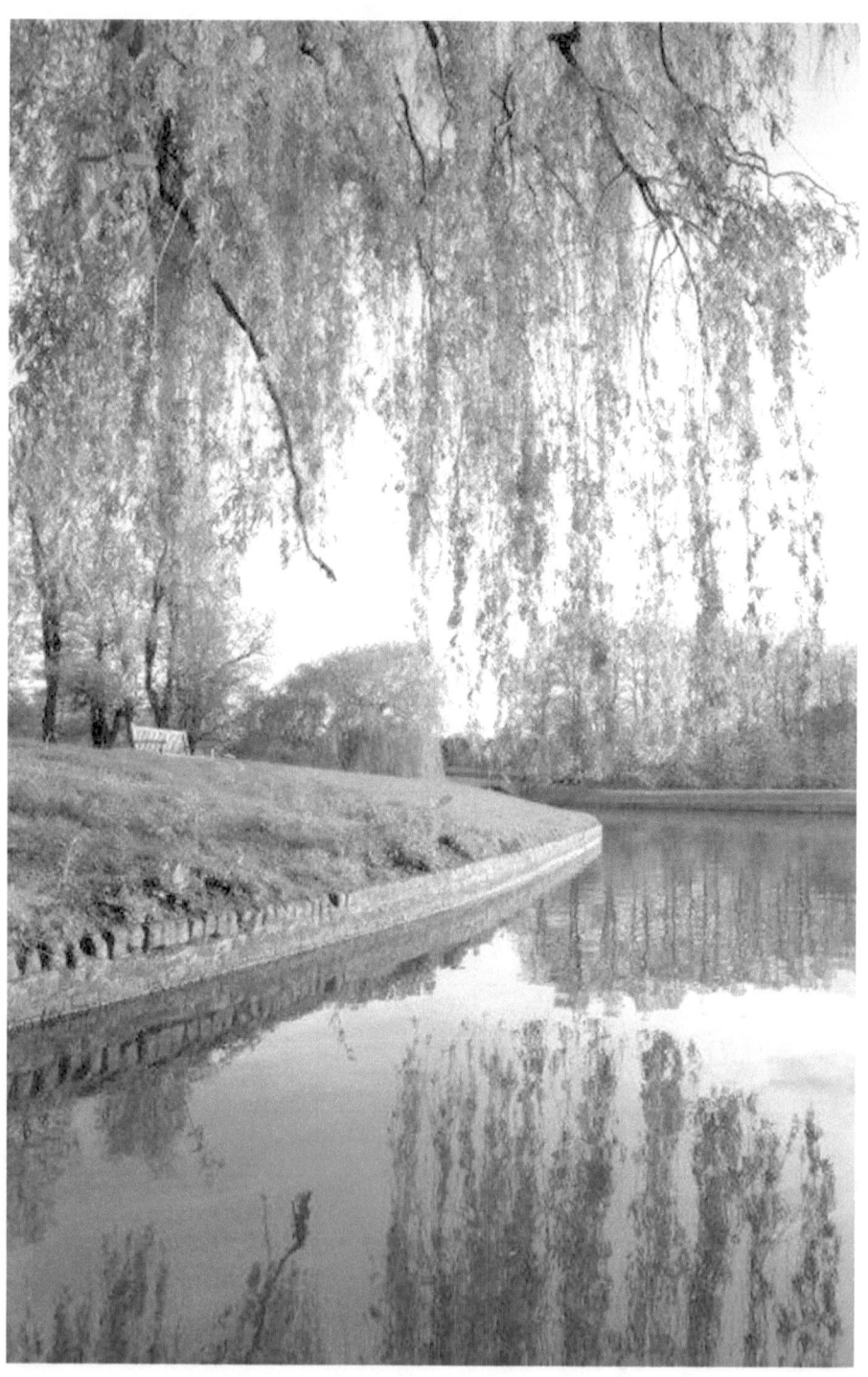

HYPERTENSION DIARY AND LOG

BLOOD PRESSURE LOG

Date / Day	Time	AM	PM	SYSTOLIC	DIASTOLIC	Pulse Rate

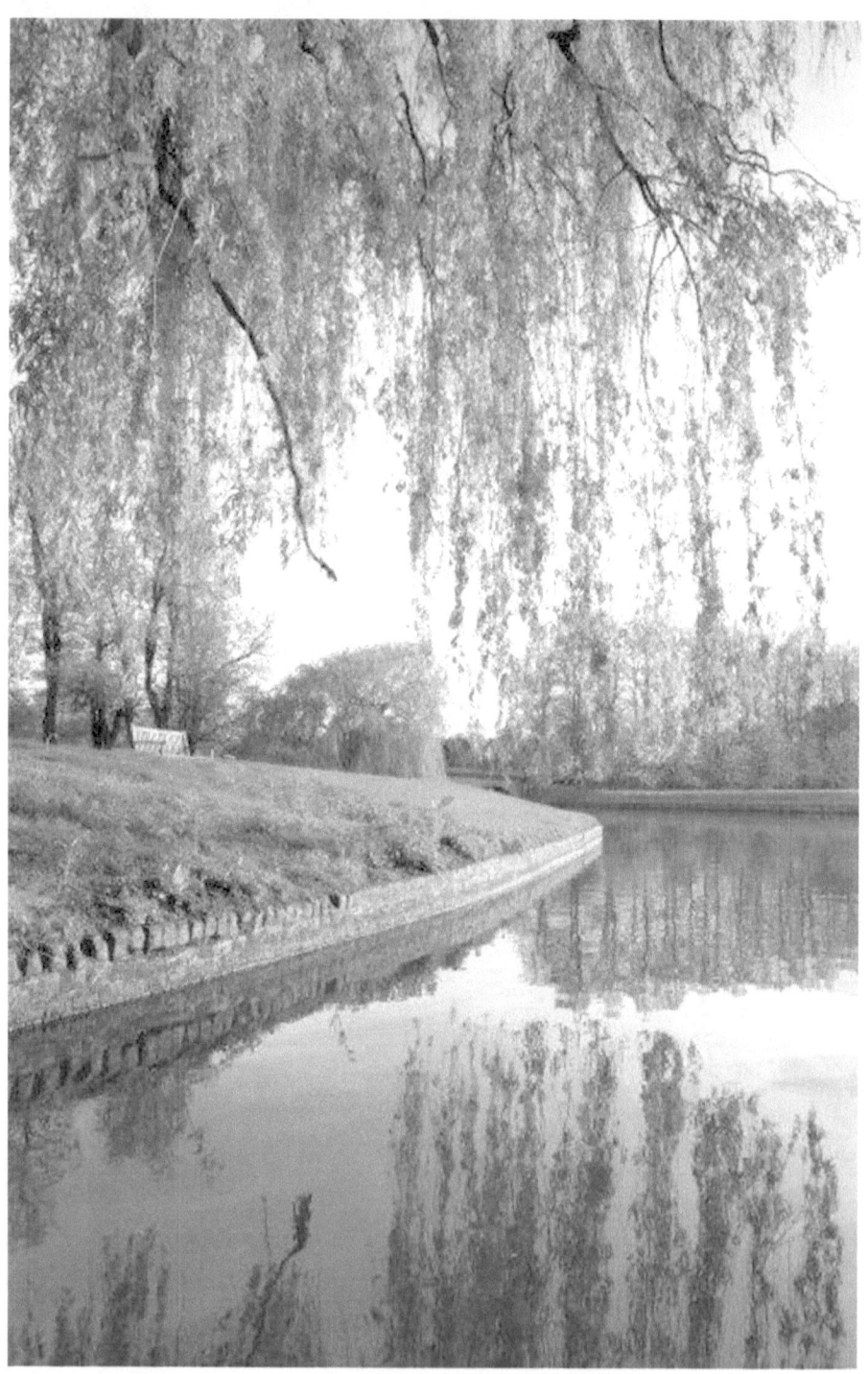

HYPERTENSION DIARY AND LOG

BLOOD PRESSURE LOG

Date / Day	Time	AM	PM	SYSTOLIC	DIASTOLIC	Pulse Rate

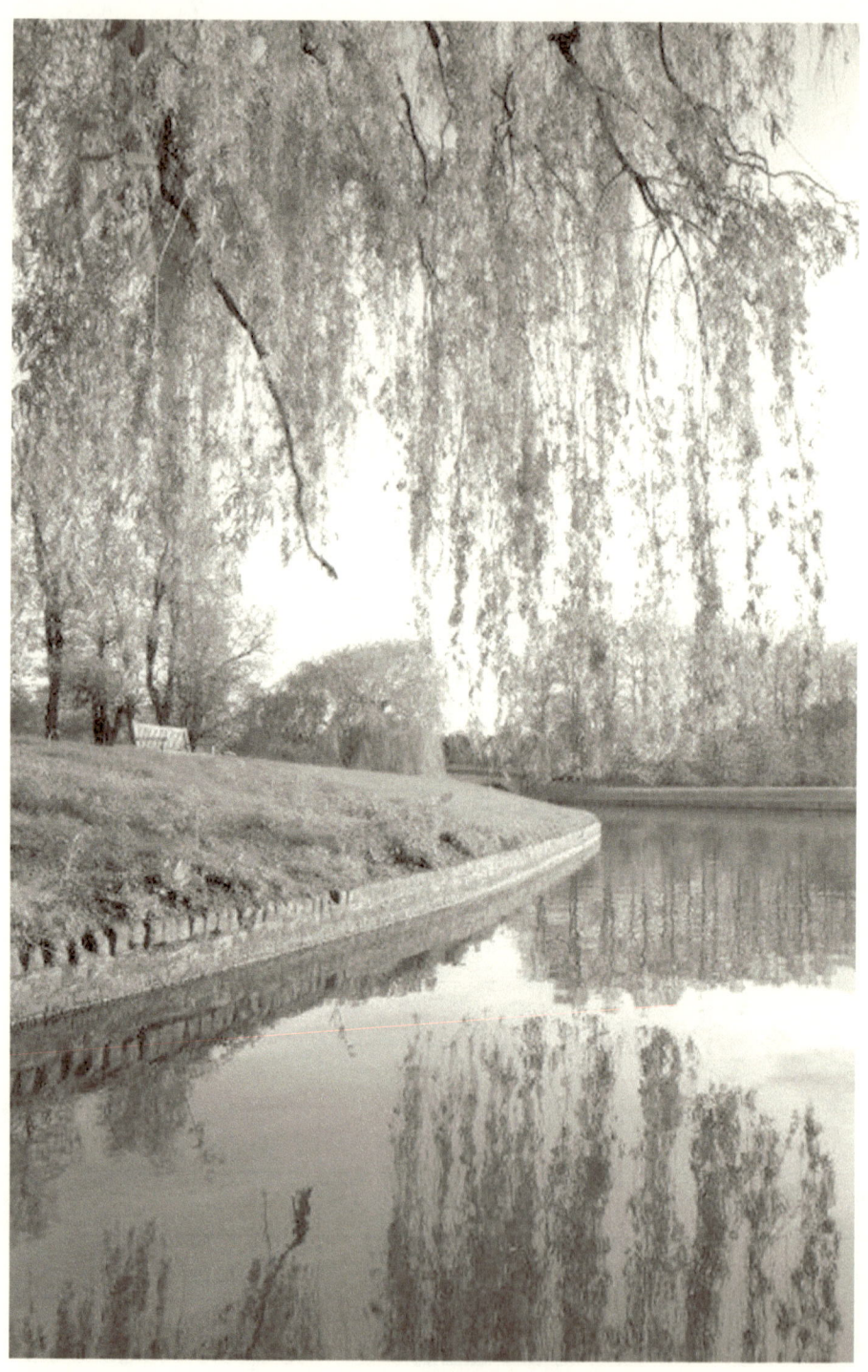

BLOOD PRESSURE LOG

Date / Day	Time	AM	PM	SYSTOLIC	DIASTOLIC	Pulse Rate

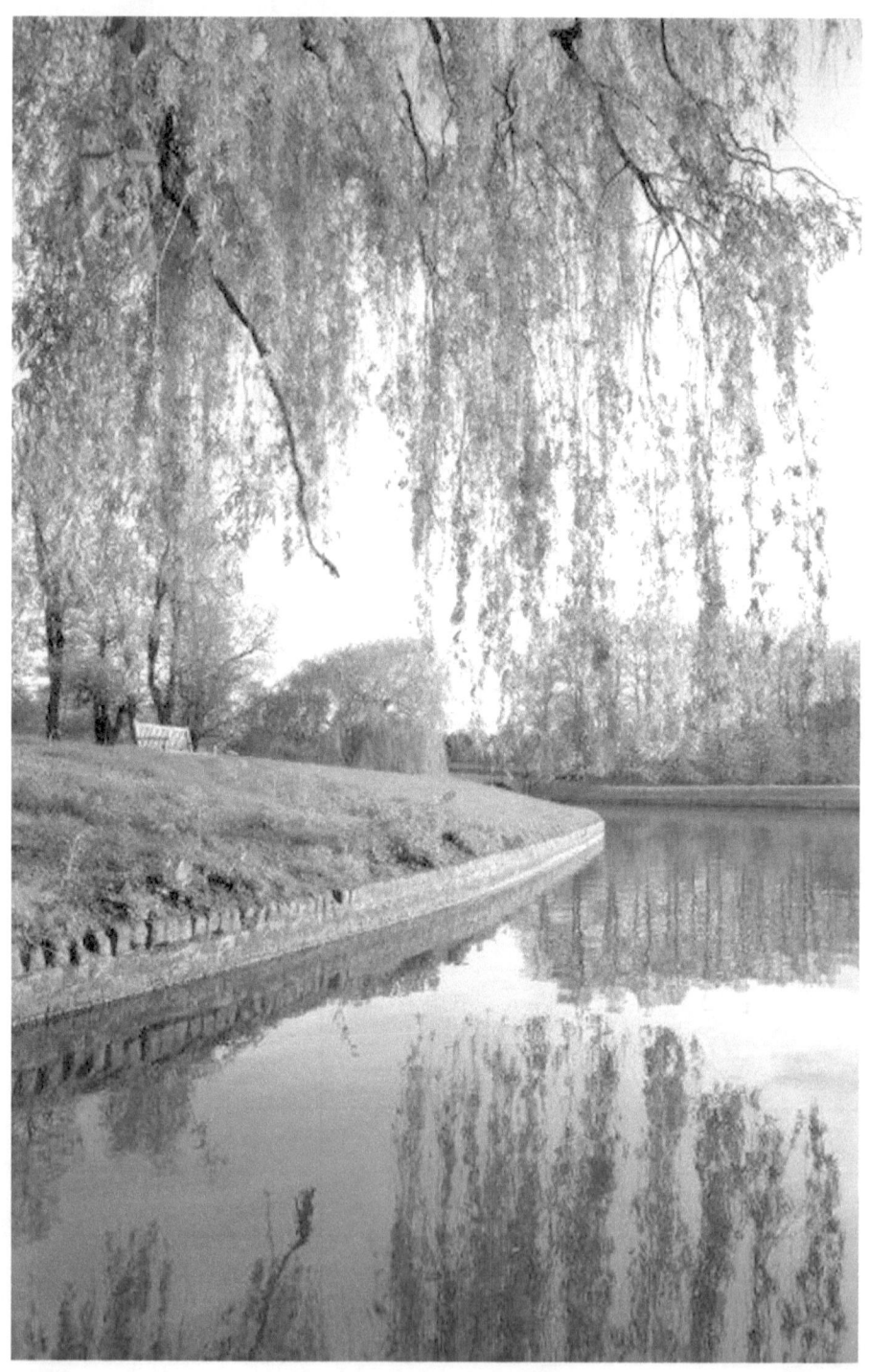

HYPERTENSION DIARY AND LOG

BLOOD PRESSURE LOG

Date / Day	Time	AM	PM	SYSTOLIC	DIASTOLIC	Pulse Rate

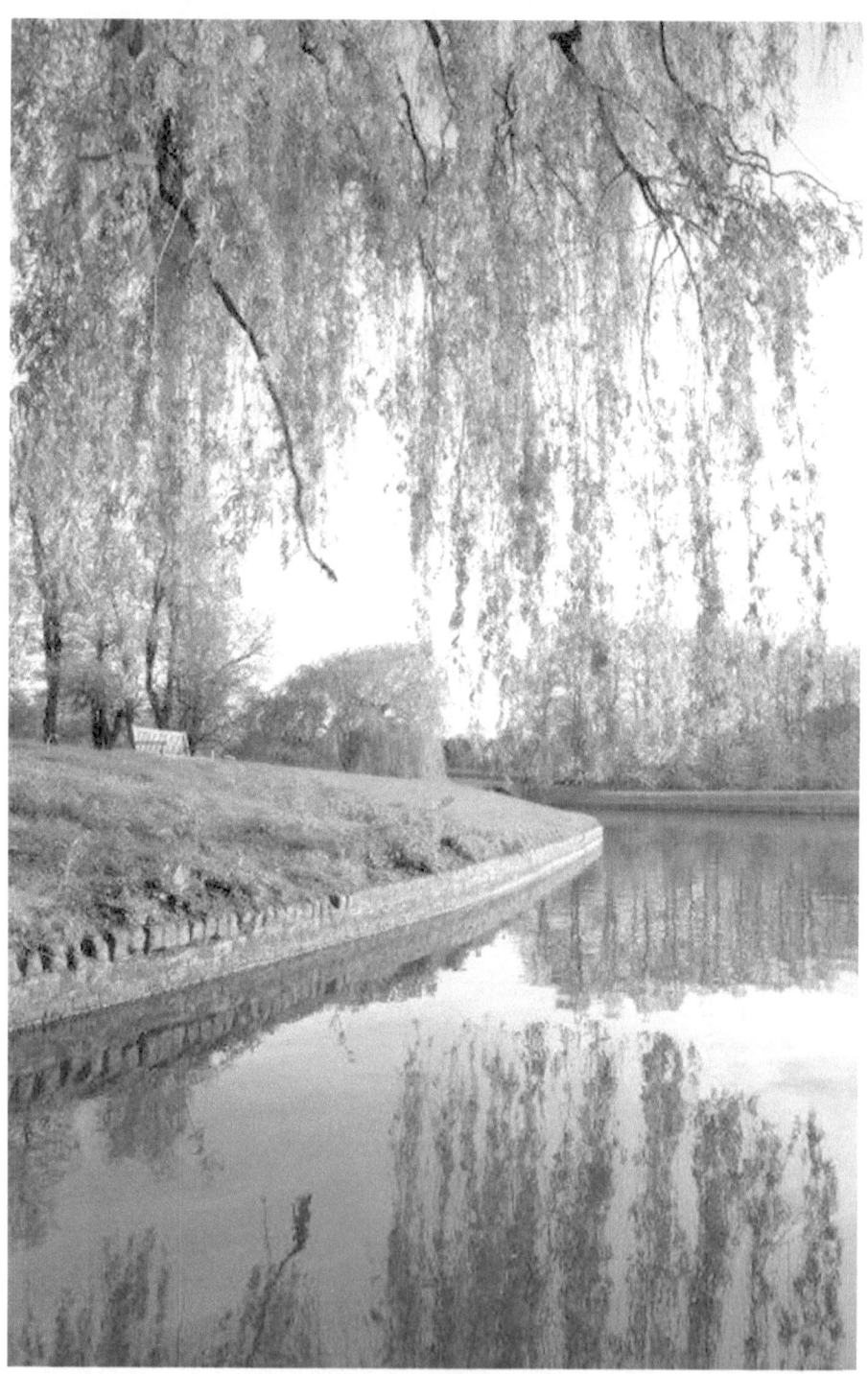

HYPERTENSION DIARY AND LOG

BLOOD PRESSURE LOG

Date / Day	Time	AM	PM	SYSTOLIC	DIASTOLIC	Pulse Rate

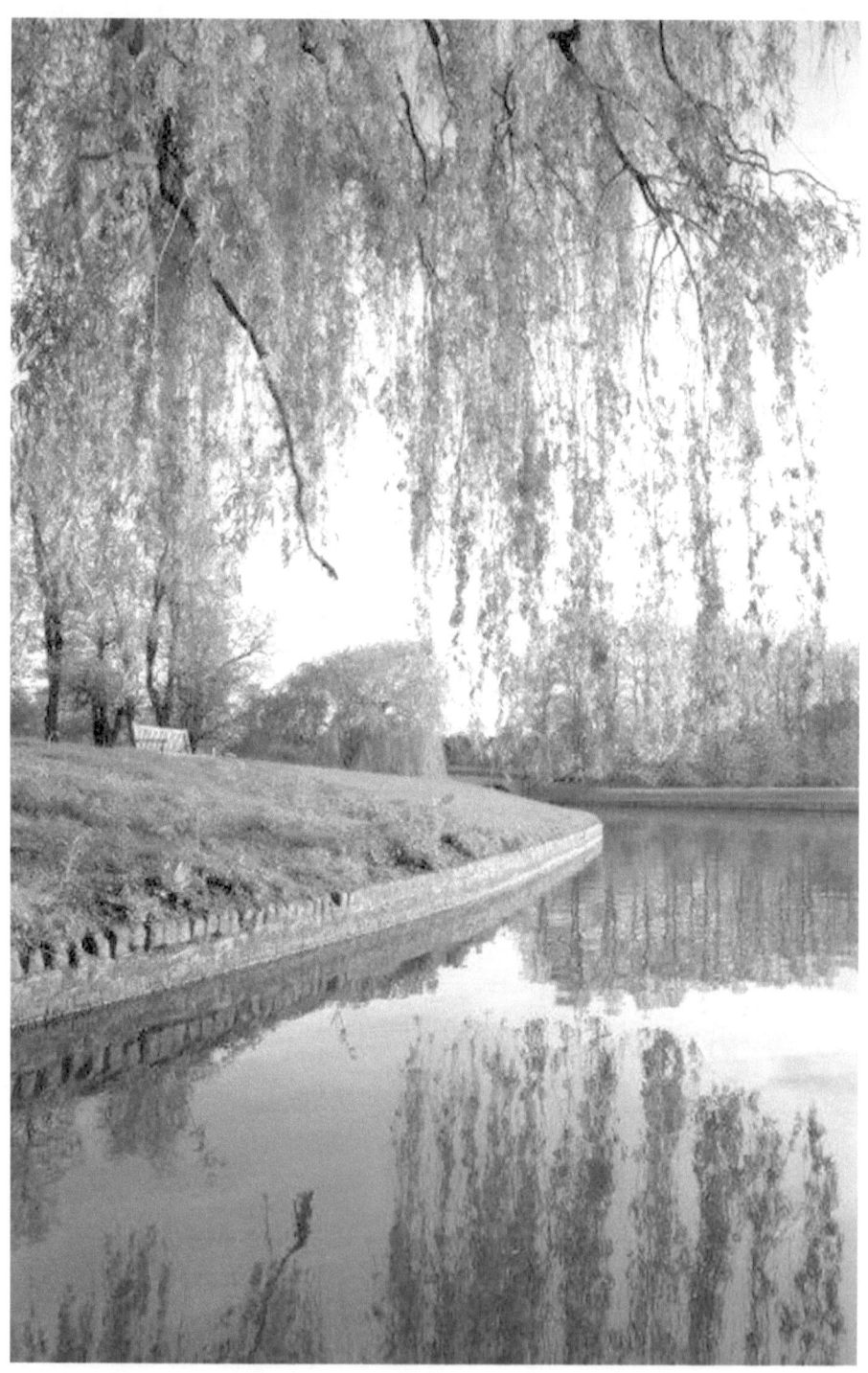

BLOOD PRESSURE LOG

Date / Day	Time	AM	PM	SYSTOLIC	DIASTOLIC	Pulse Rate

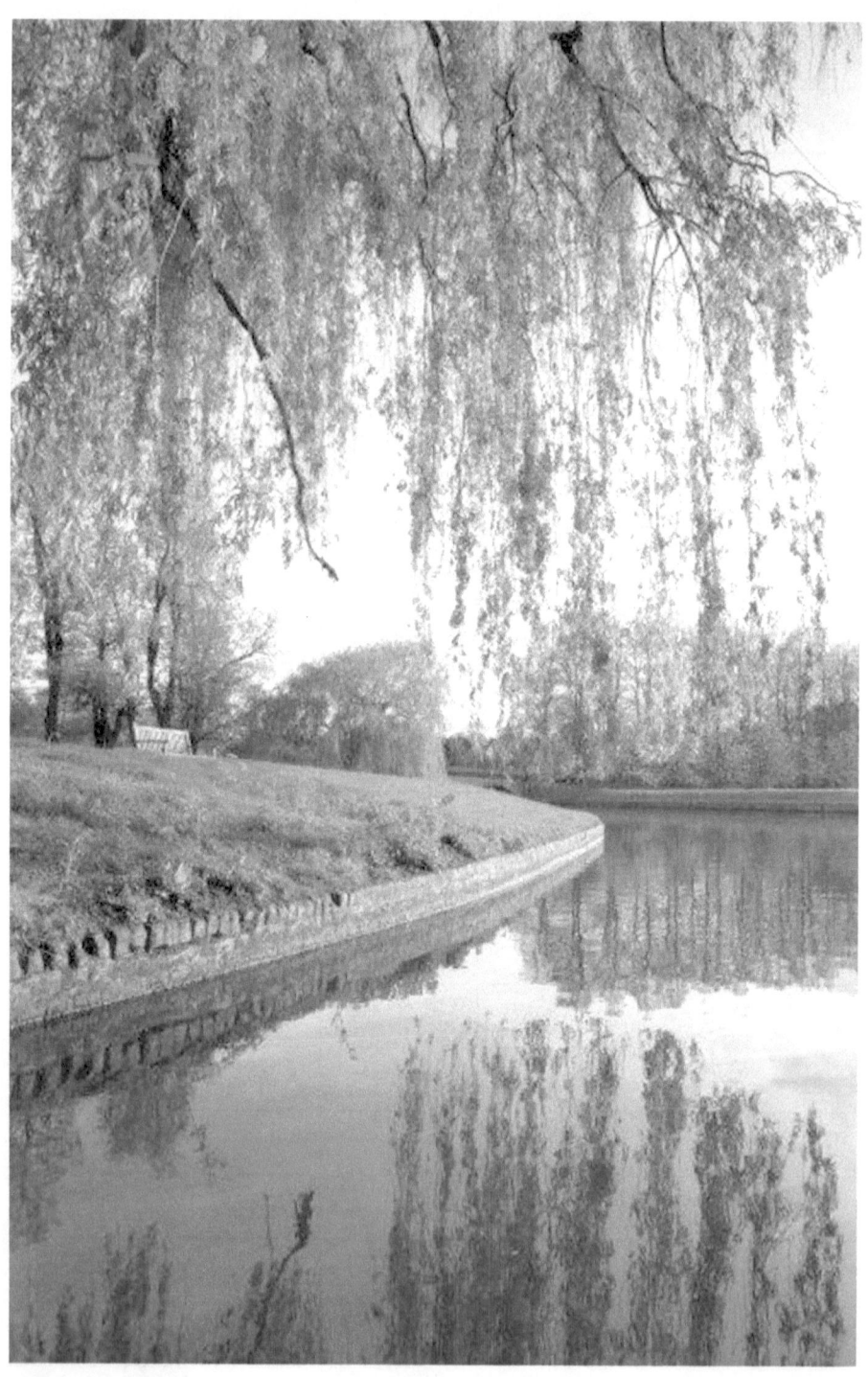

HYPERTENSION DIARY AND LOG

BLOOD PRESSURE LOG

Date / Day	Time	AM	PM	SYSTOLIC	DIASTOLIC	Pulse Rate

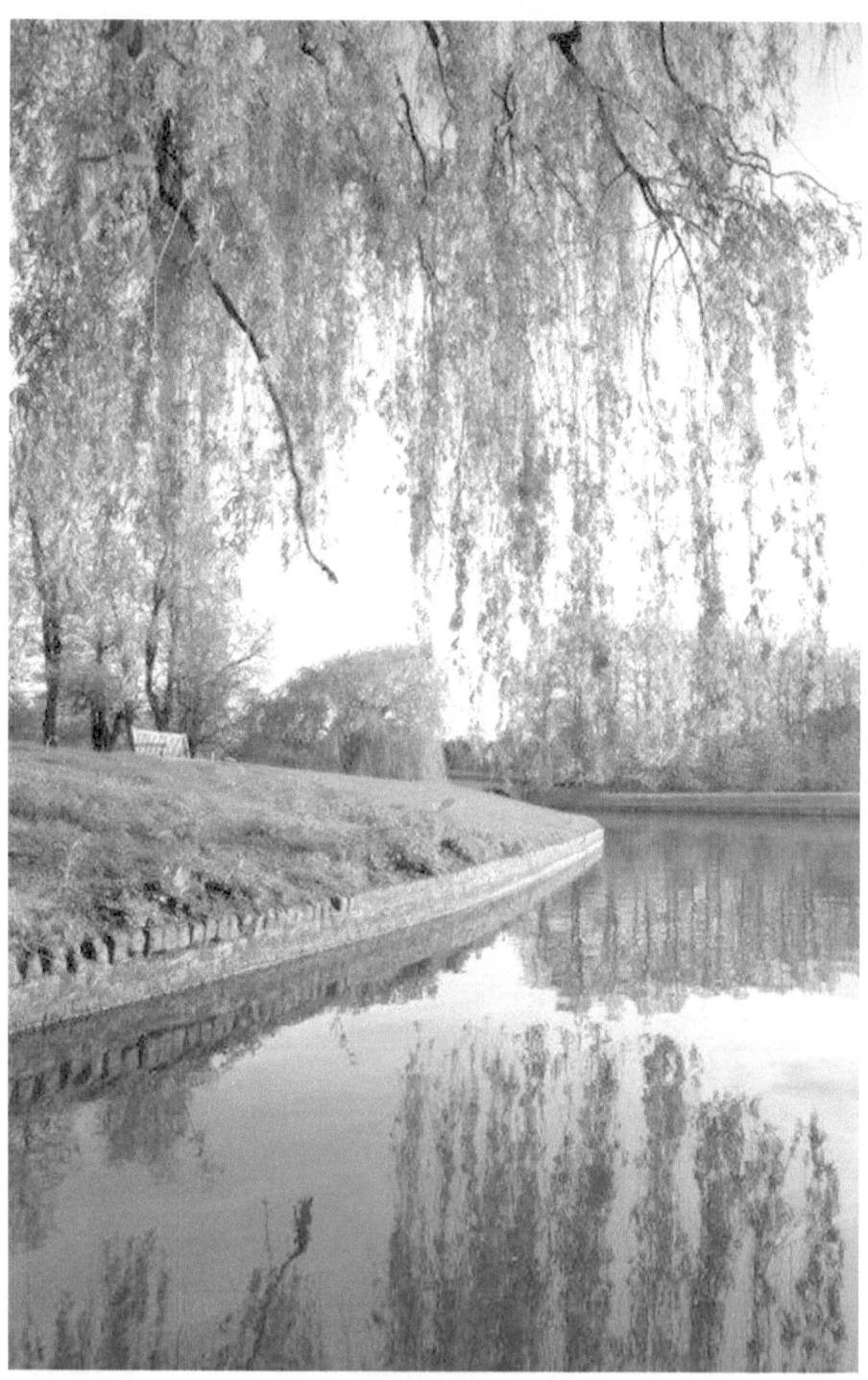

HYPERTENSION DIARY AND LOG

BLOOD PRESSURE LOG

Date / Day	Time	AM	PM	SYSTOLIC	DIASTOLIC	Pulse Rate

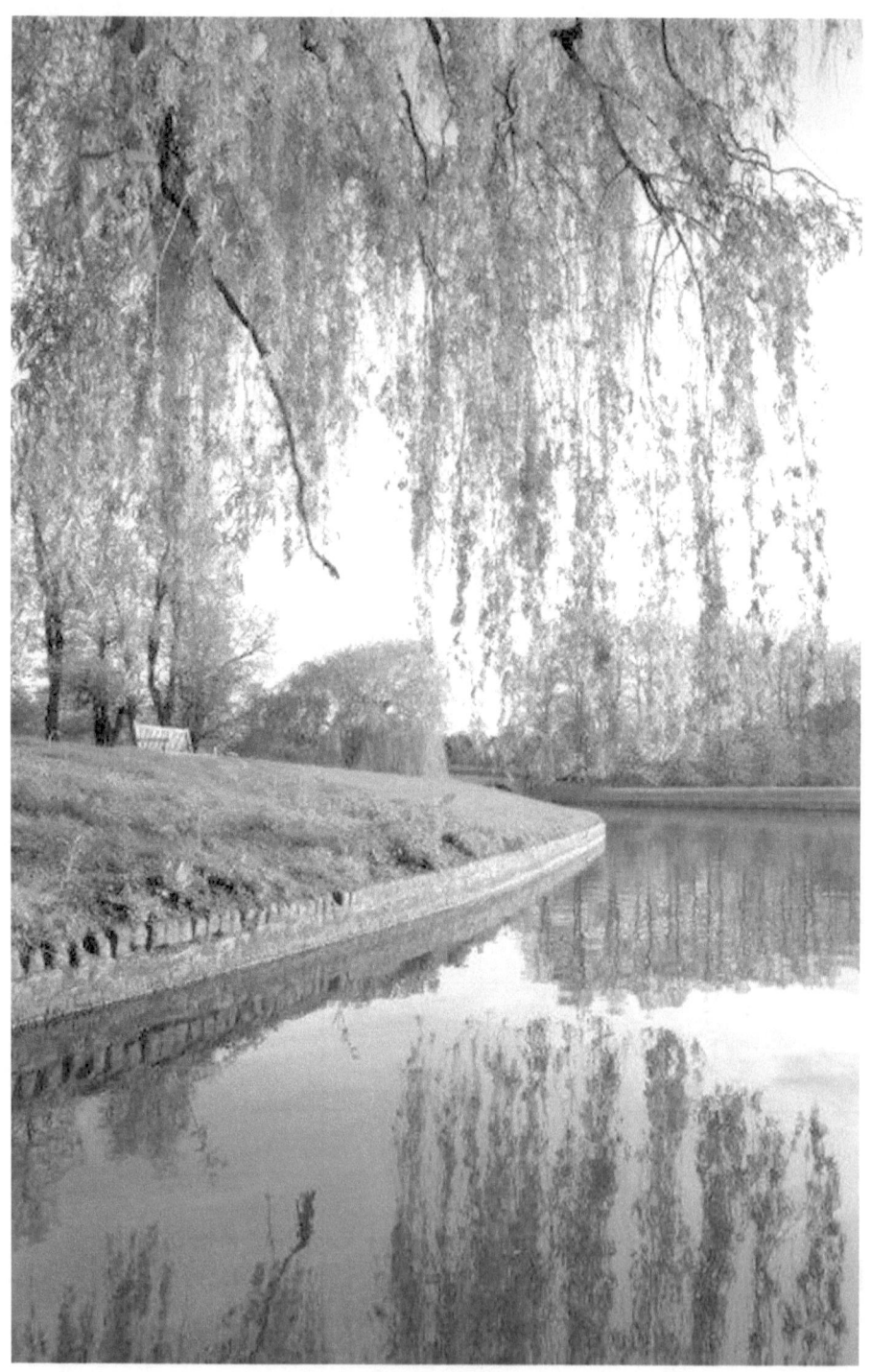

HYPERTENSION DIARY AND LOG

BLOOD PRESSURE LOG

Date / Day	Time	AM	PM	SYSTOLIC	DIASTOLIC	Pulse Rate

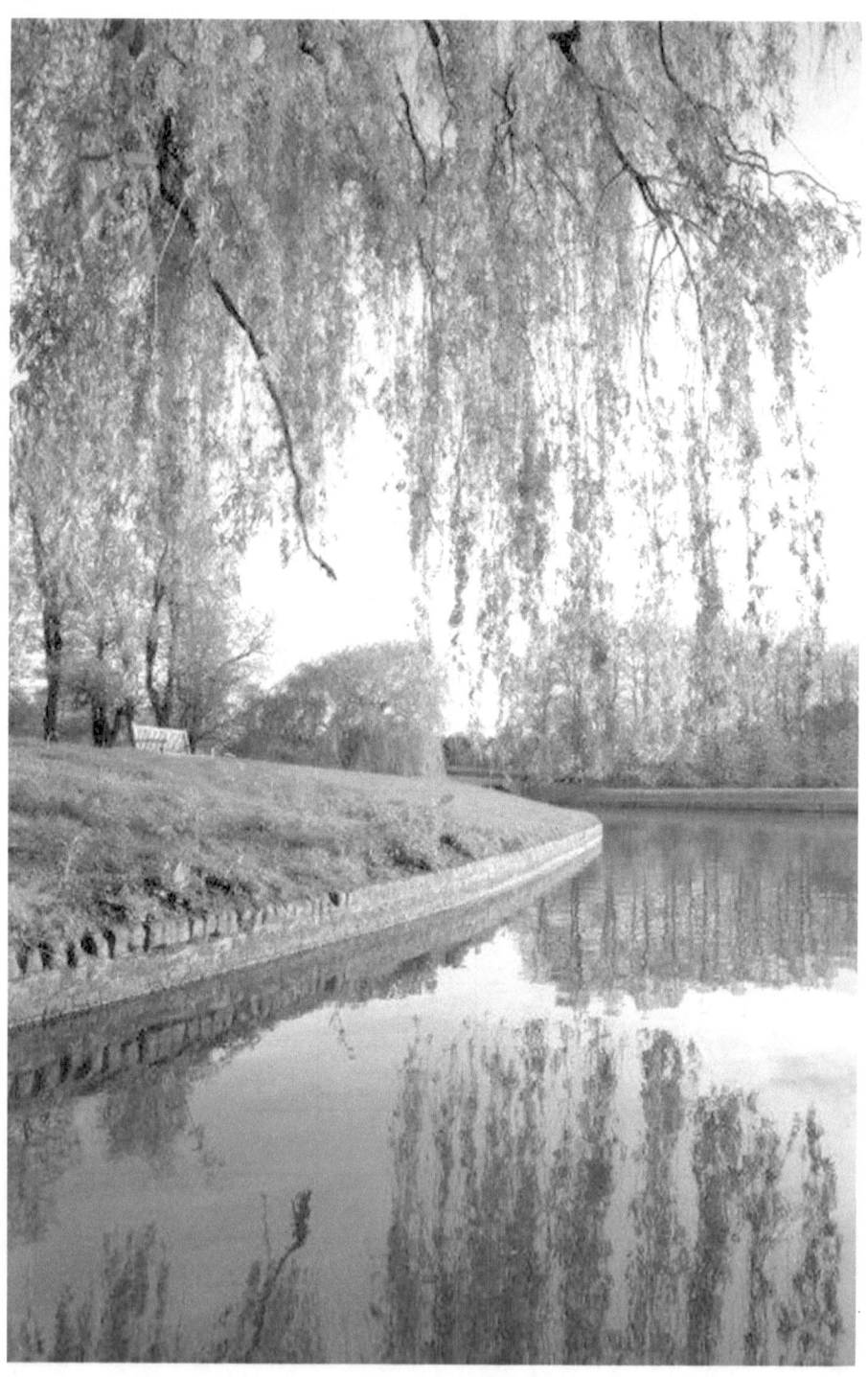

HYPERTENSION DIARY AND LOG

BLOOD PRESSURE LOG

Date / Day	Time	AM	PM	SYSTOLIC	DIASTOLIC	Pulse Rate

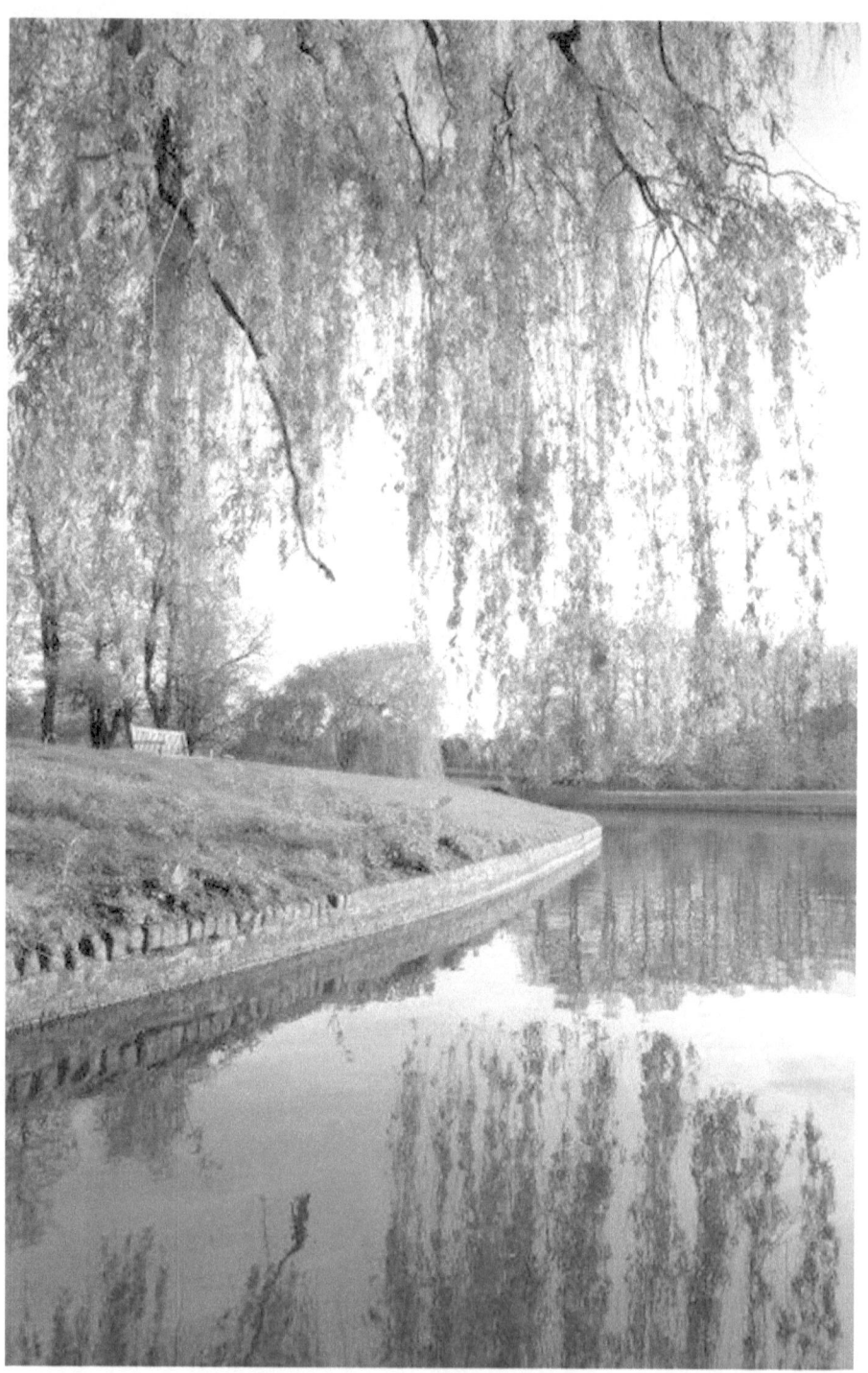

HYPERTENSION DIARY AND LOG

BLOOD PRESSURE LOG

Date / Day	Time	AM	PM	SYSTOLIC	DIASTOLIC	Pulse Rate

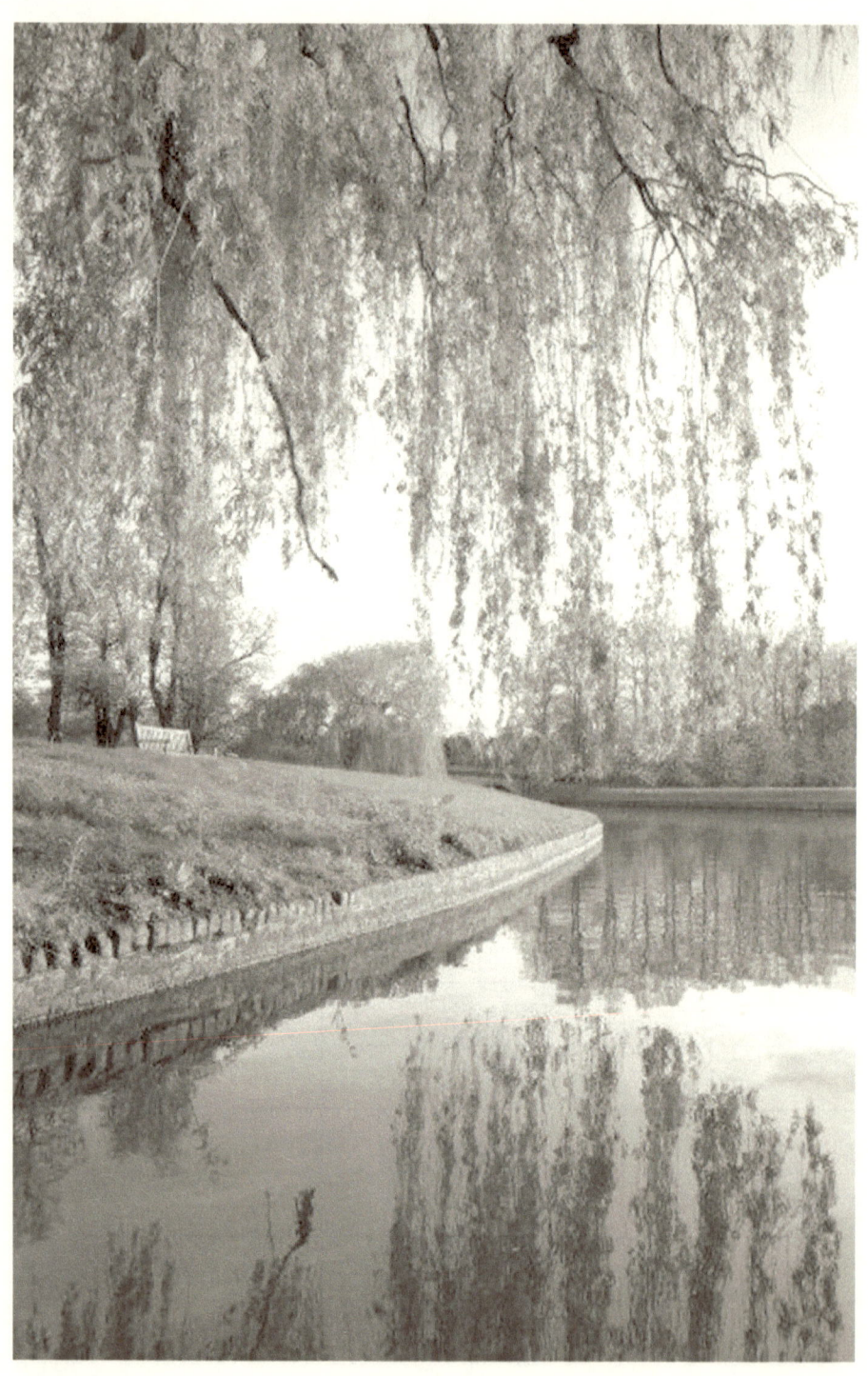

BLOOD PRESSURE LOG

Date / Day	Time	AM	PM	SYSTOLIC	DIASTOLIC	Pulse Rate

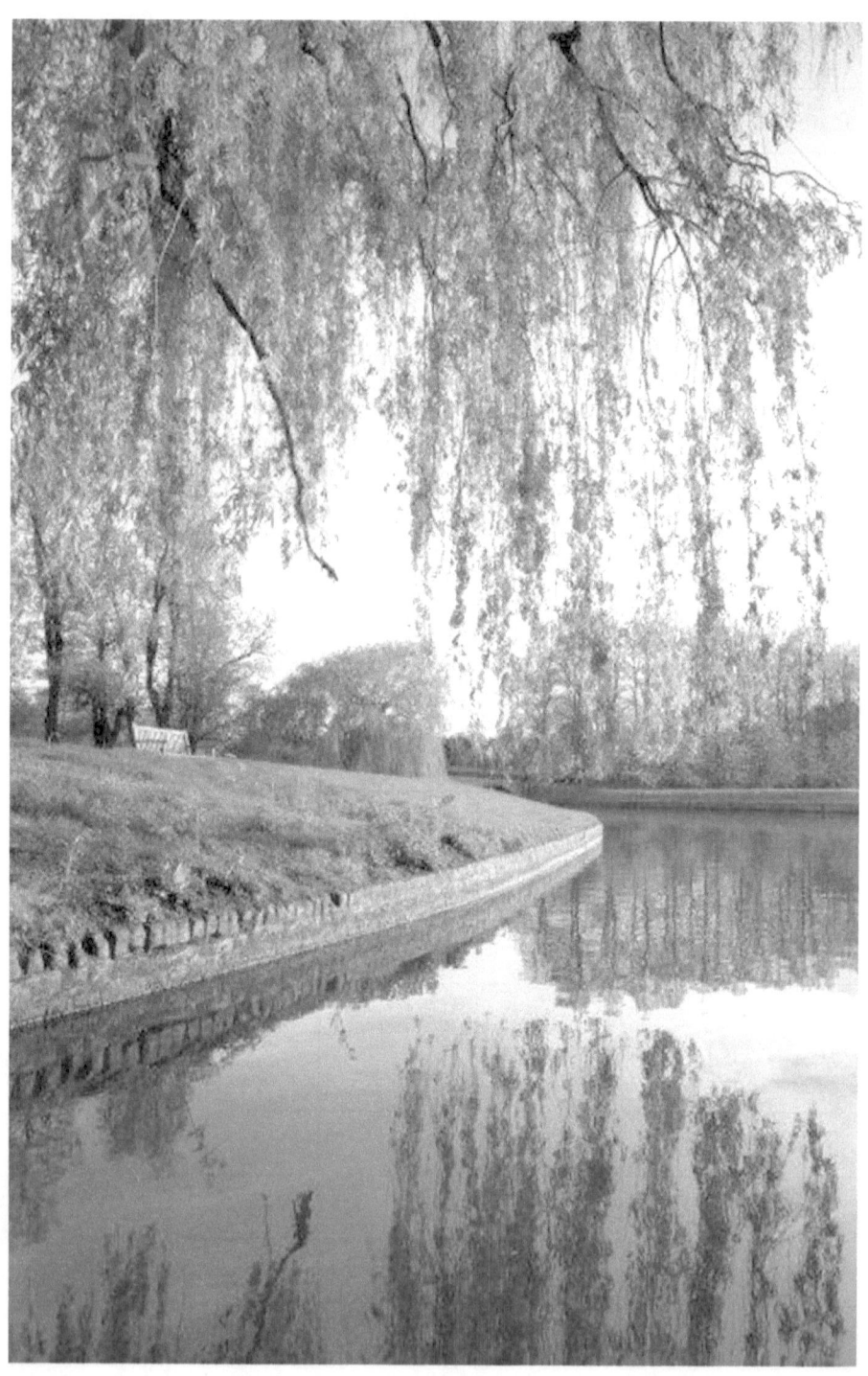

HYPERTENSION DIARY AND LOG

BLOOD PRESSURE LOG

Date / Day	Time	AM	PM	SYSTOLIC	DIASTOLIC	Pulse Rate

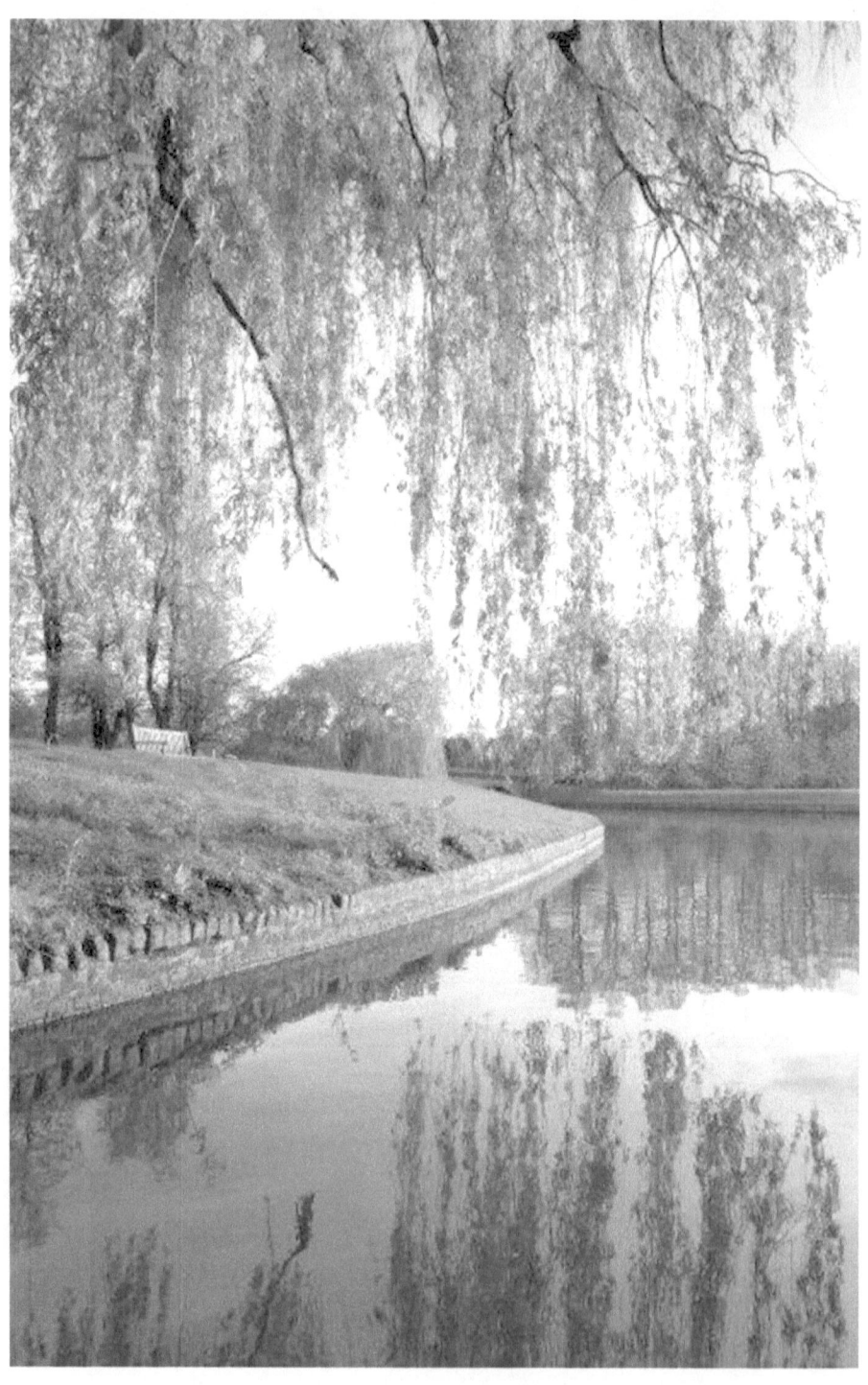

HYPERTENSION DIARY AND LOG

BLOOD PRESSURE LOG

Date / Day	Time	AM	PM	SYSTOLIC	DIASTOLIC	Pulse Rate

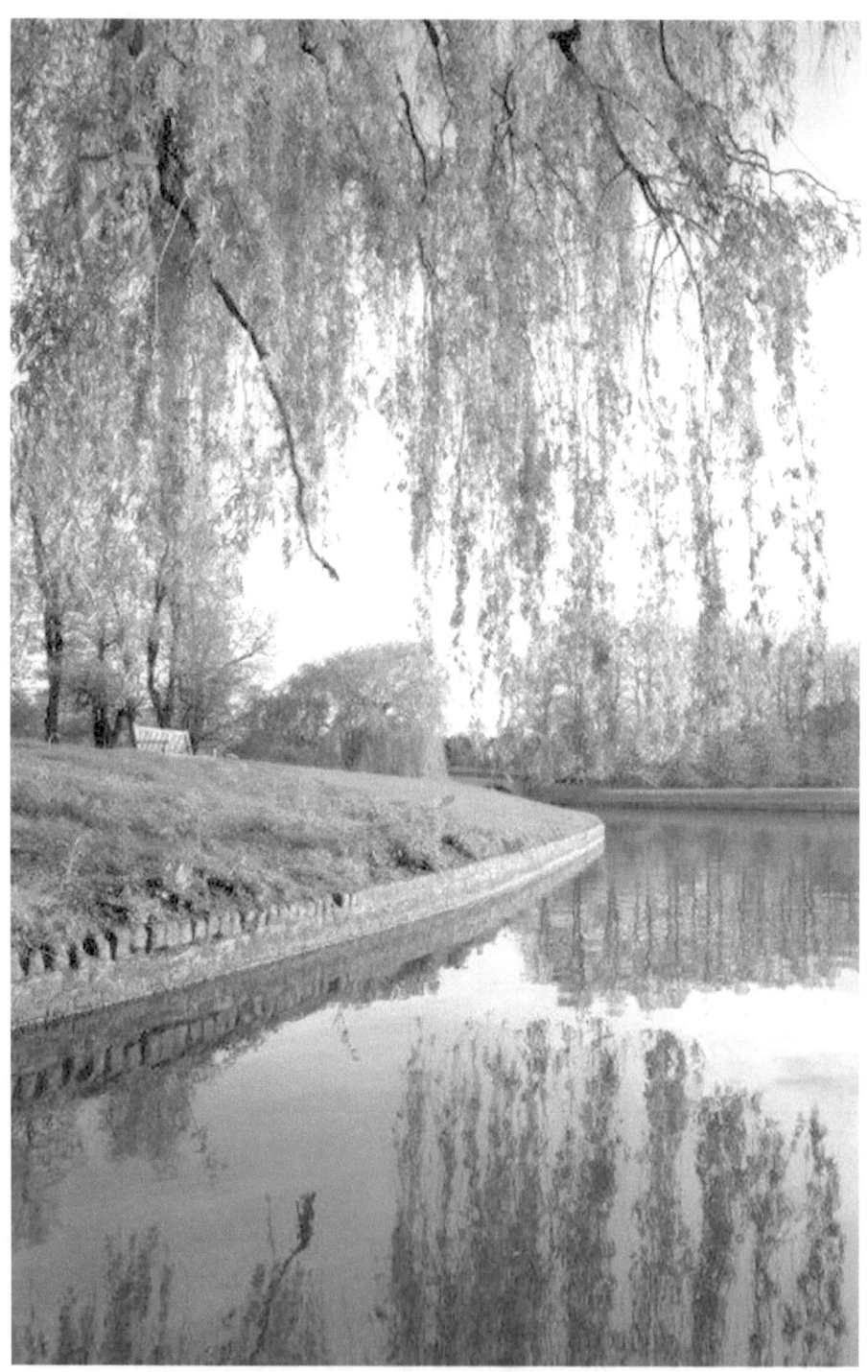

HYPERTENSION DIARY AND LOG

BLOOD PRESSURE LOG

Date / Day	Time	AM	PM	SYSTOLIC	DIASTOLIC	Pulse Rate

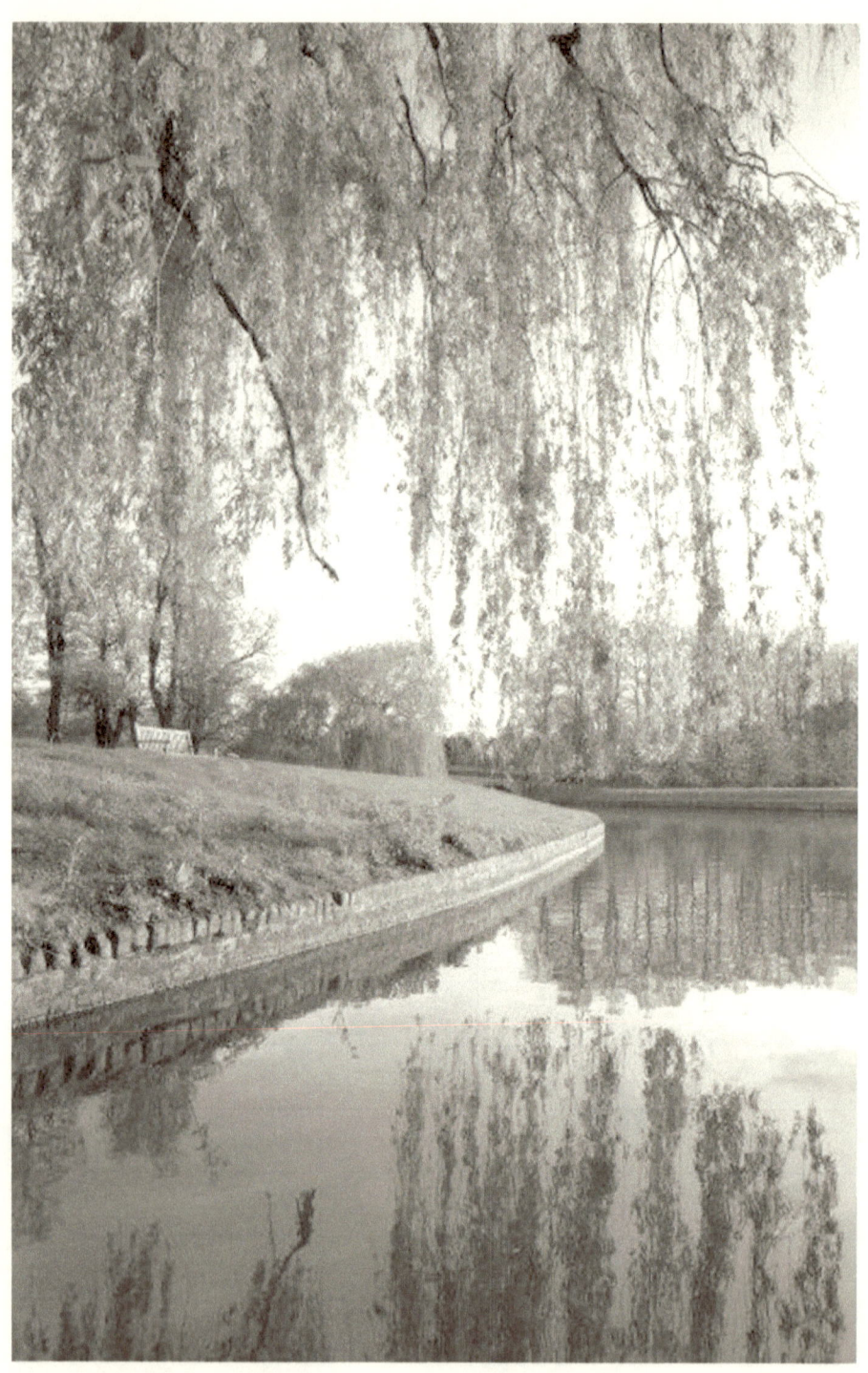

HYPERTENSION DIARY AND LOG

BLOOD PRESSURE LOG

Date / Day	Time	AM	PM	SYSTOLIC	DIASTOLIC	Pulse Rate

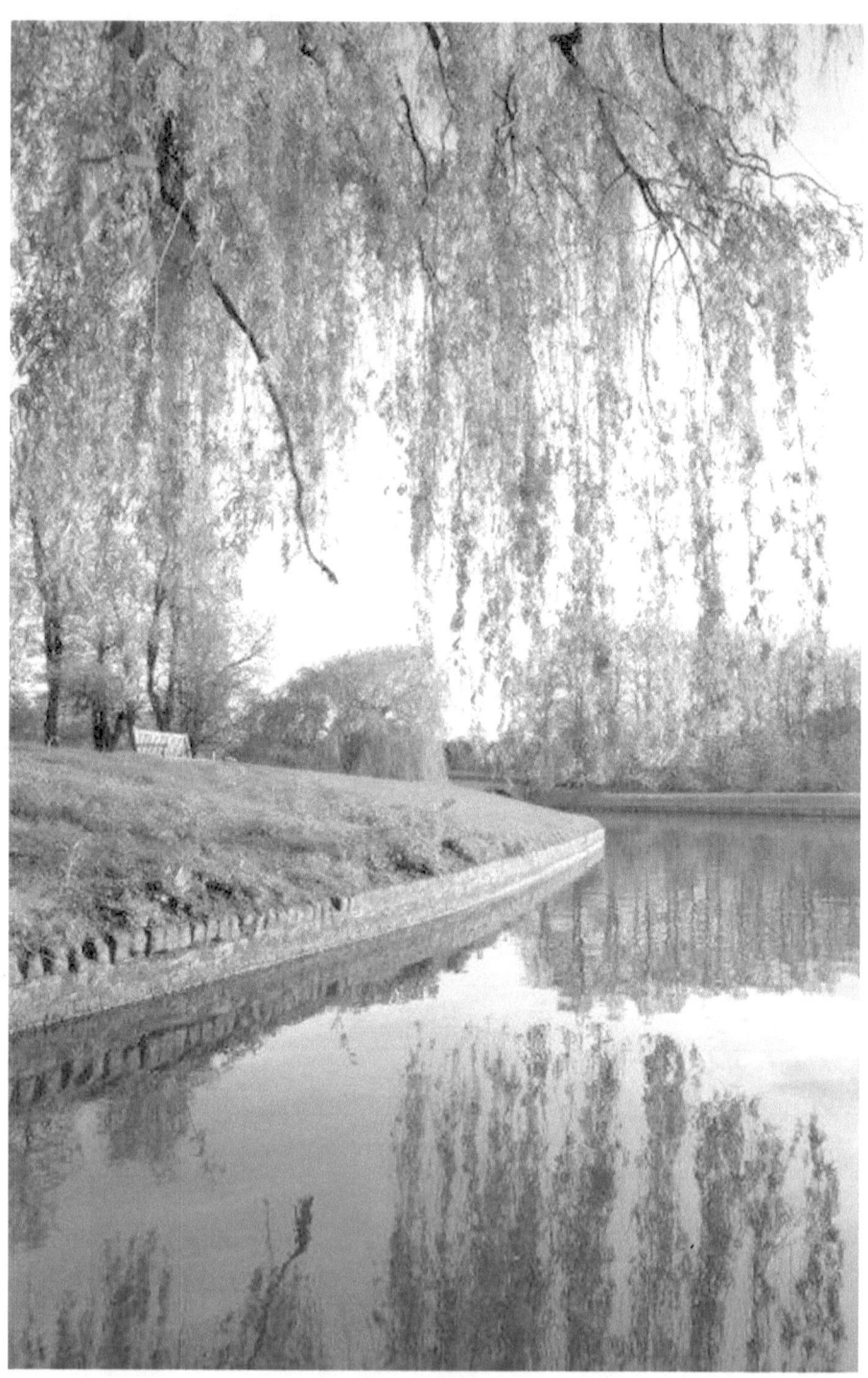

HYPERTENSION DIARY AND LOG

BLOOD PRESSURE LOG

Date / Day	Time	AM	PM	SYSTOLIC	DIASTOLIC	Pulse Rate

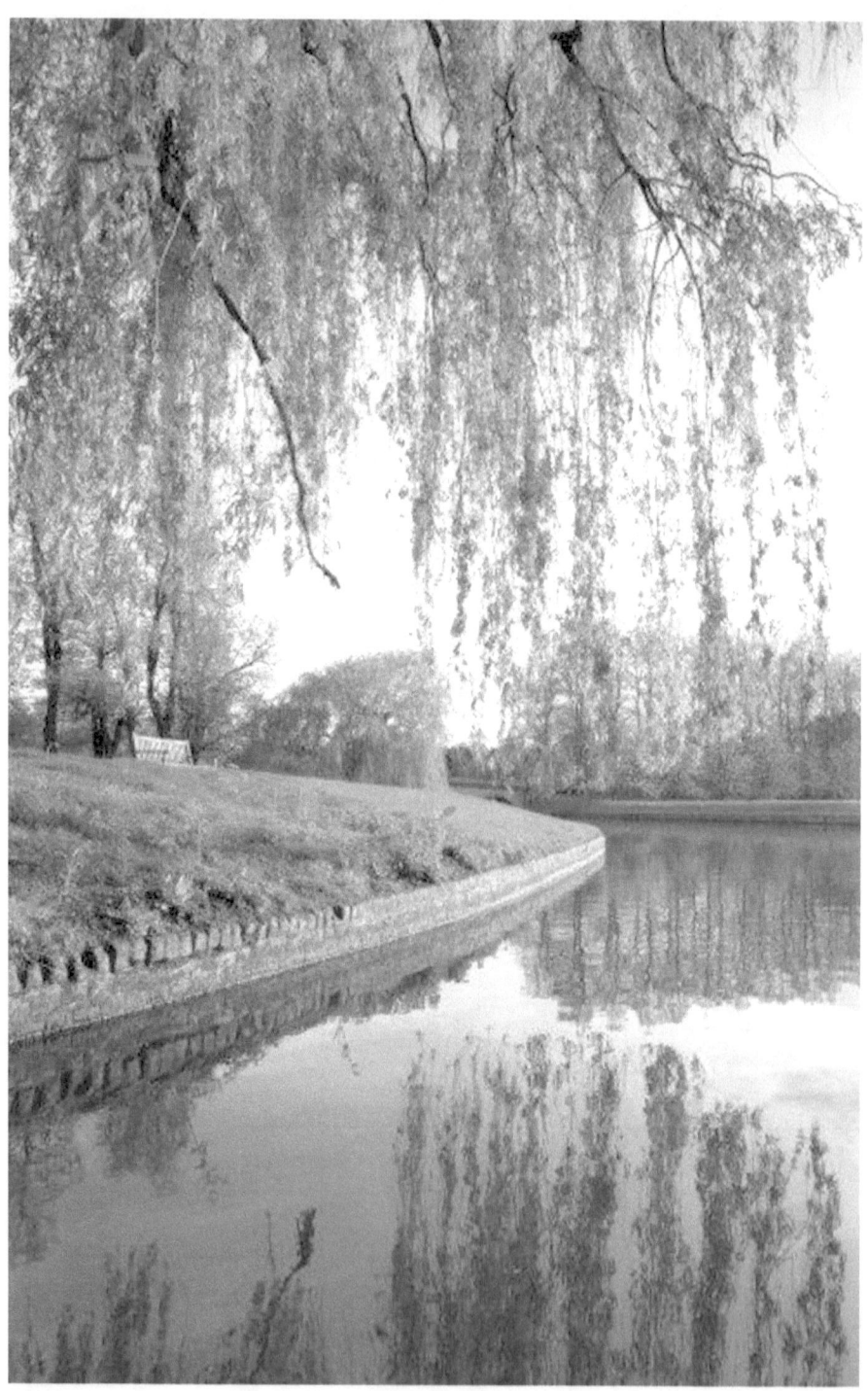

HYPERTENSION DIARY AND LOG

BLOOD PRESSURE LOG

Date / Day	Time	AM	PM	SYSTOLIC	DIASTOLIC	Pulse Rate

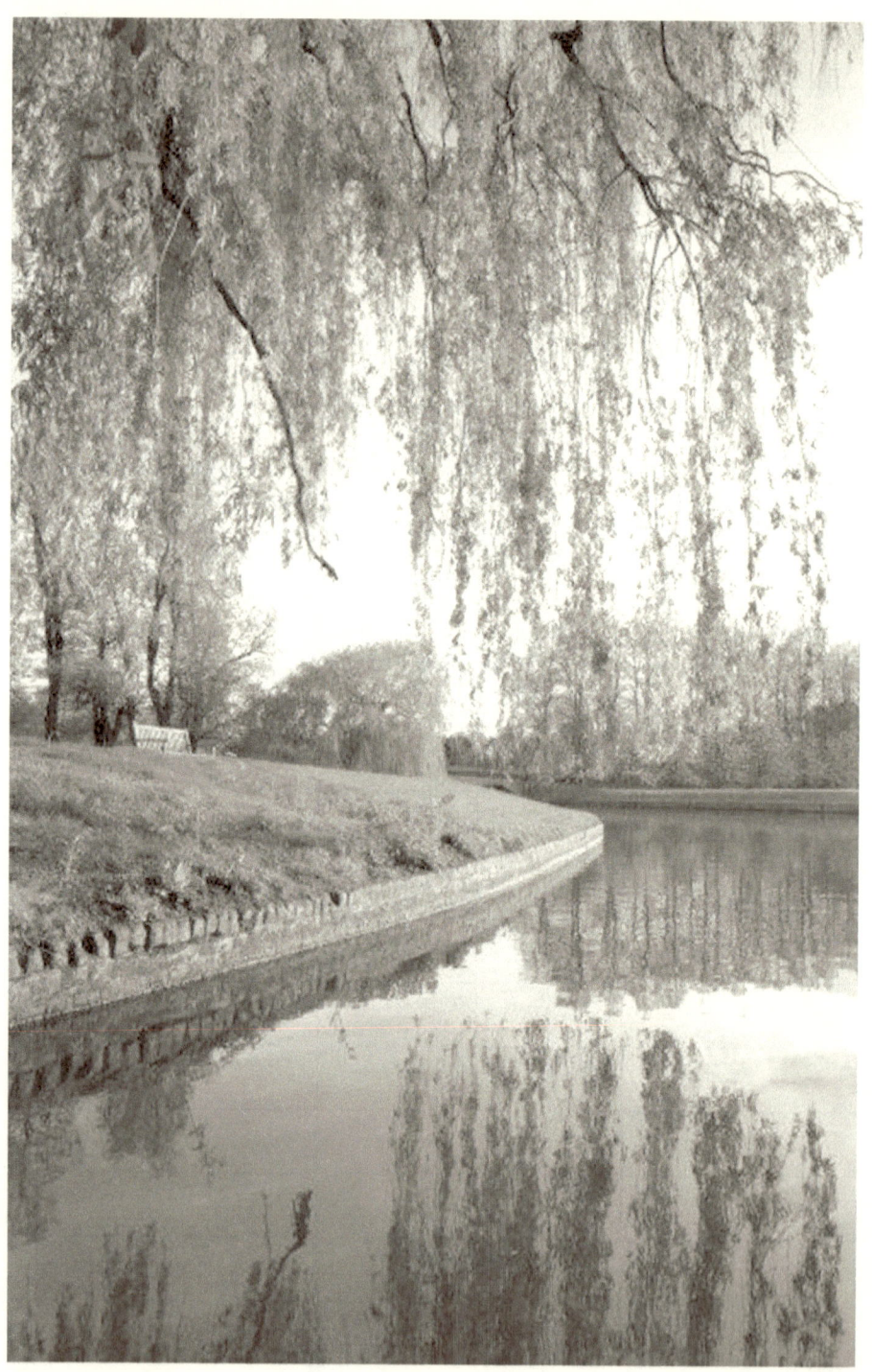

HYPERTENSION DIARY AND LOG

BLOOD PRESSURE LOG

Date / Day	Time	AM	PM	SYSTOLIC	DIASTOLIC	Pulse Rate

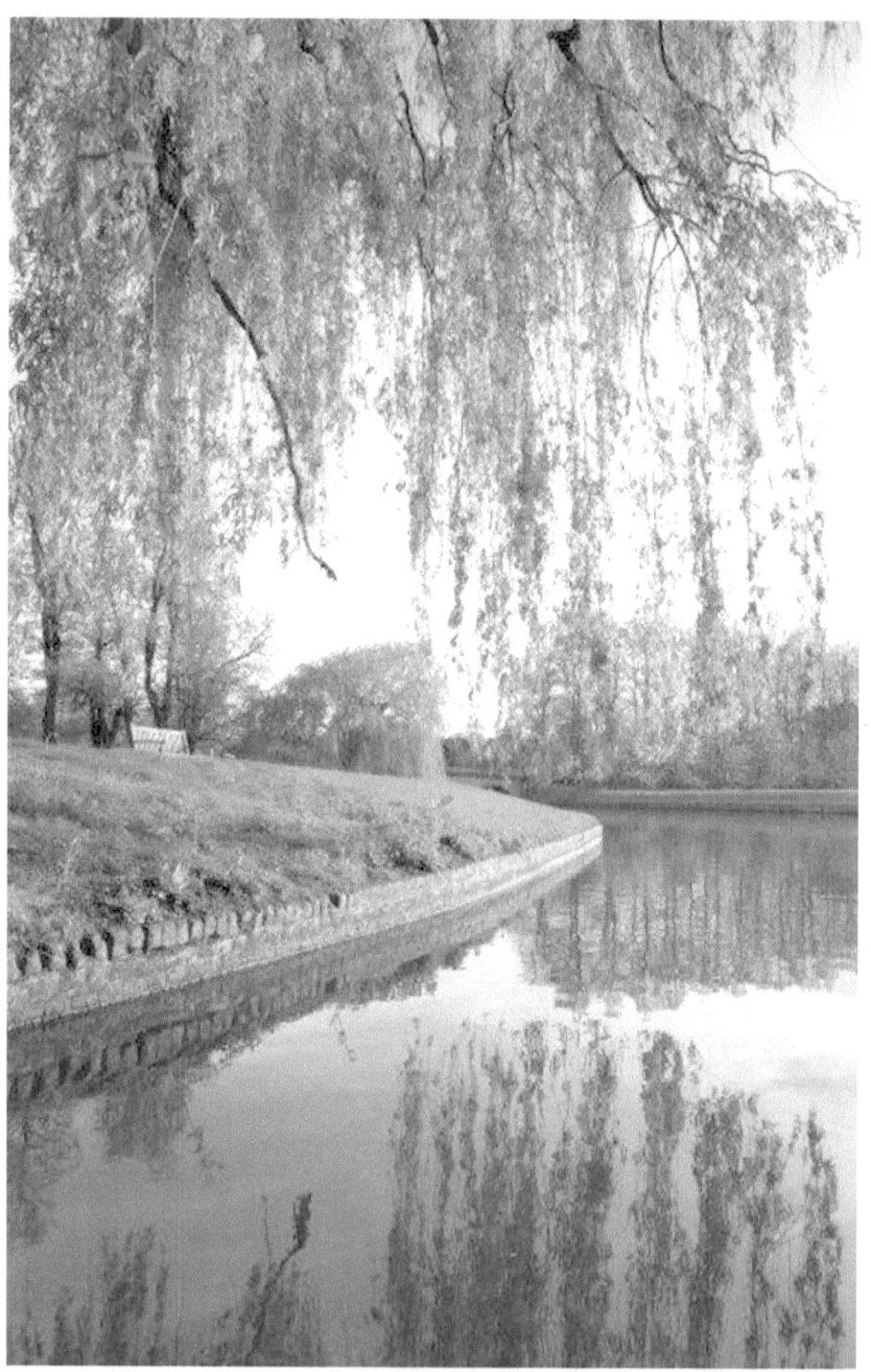

HYPERTENSION DIARY AND LOG

BLOOD PRESSURE LOG

Date / Day	Time	AM	PM	SYSTOLIC	DIASTOLIC	Pulse Rate

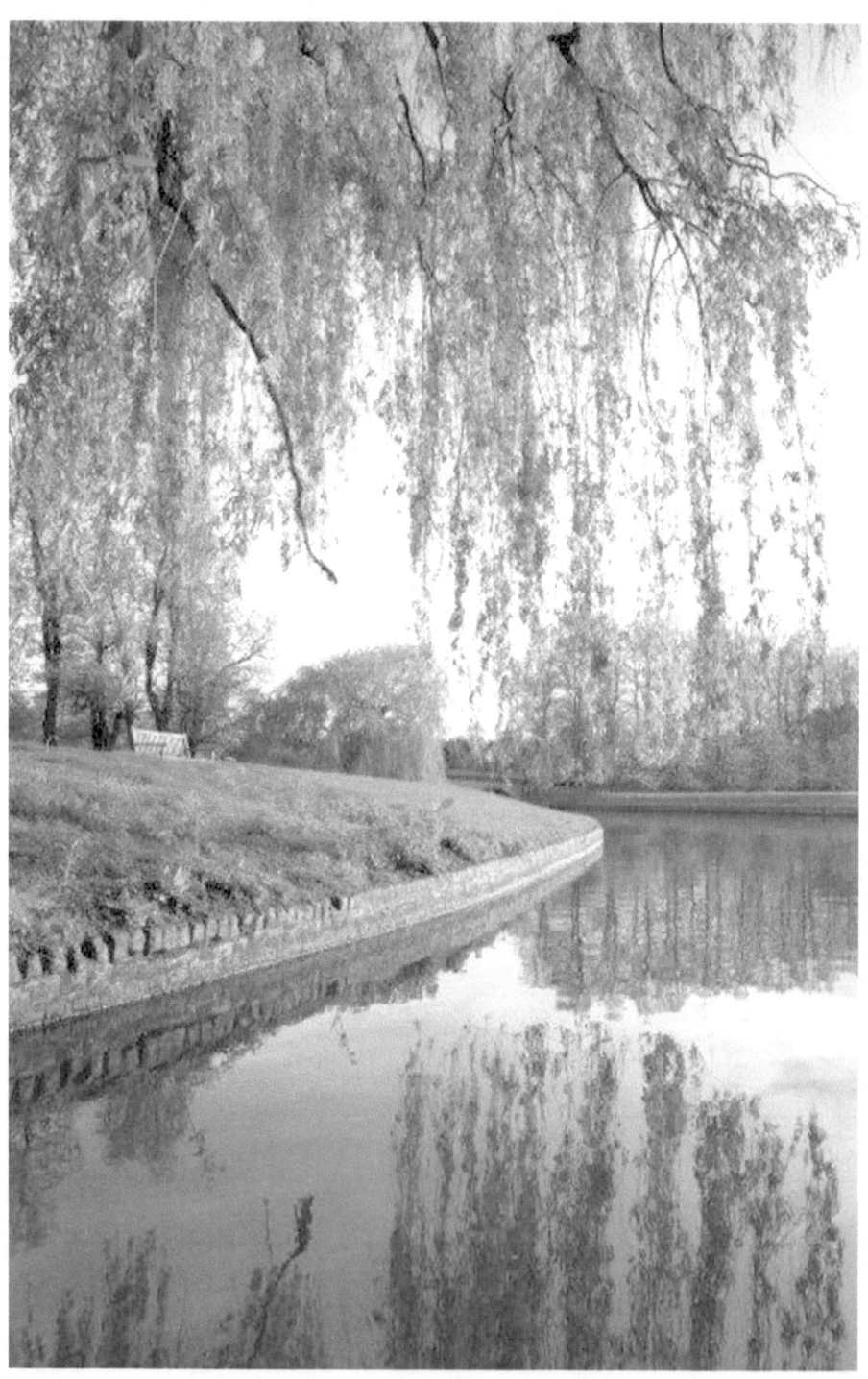

HYPERTENSION DIARY AND LOG

BLOOD PRESSURE LOG

Date / Day	Time	AM	PM	SYSTOLIC	DIASTOLIC	Pulse Rate

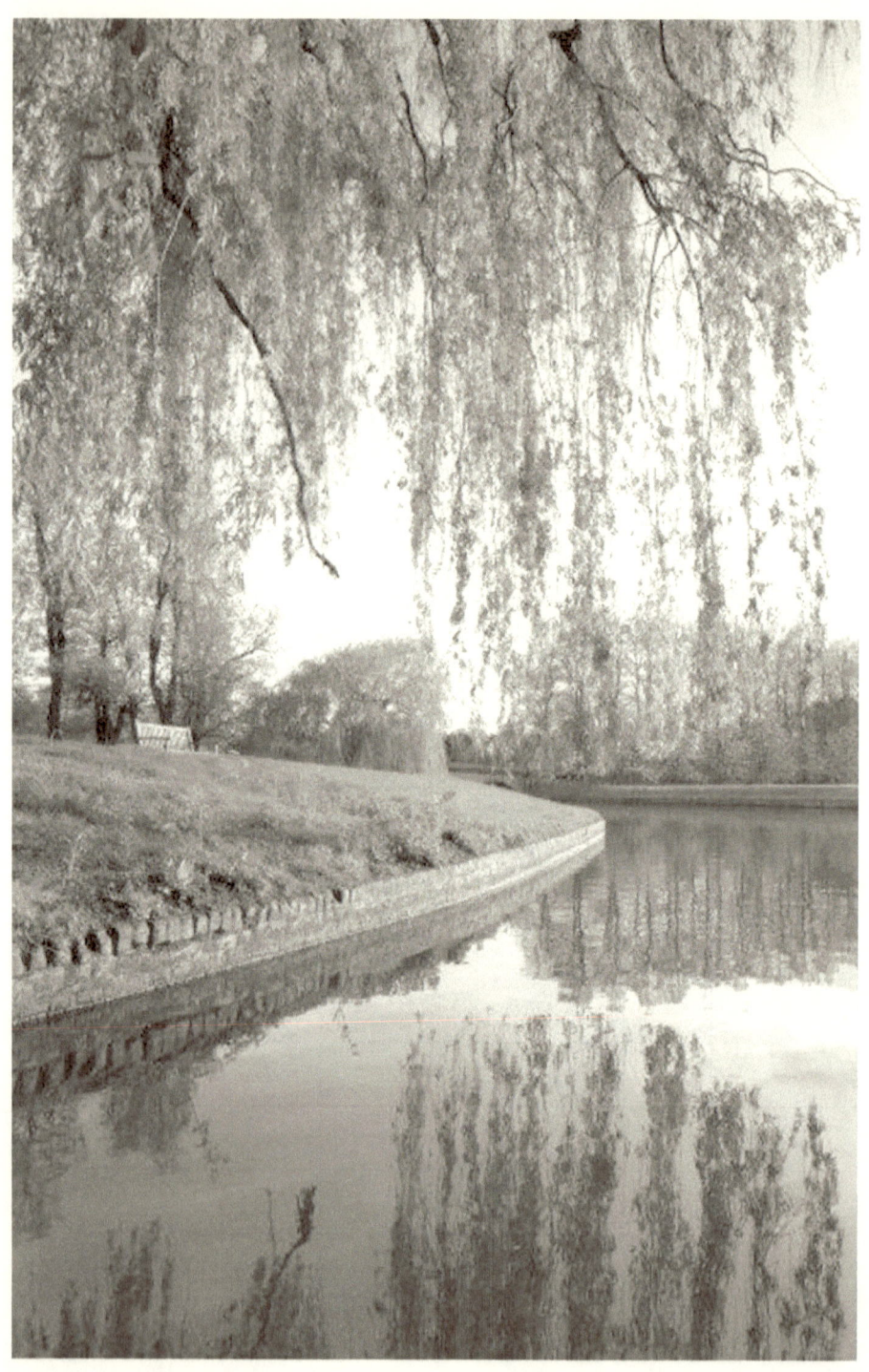

BLOOD PRESSURE LOG

Date / Day	Time	AM	PM	SYSTOLIC	DIASTOLIC	Pulse Rate

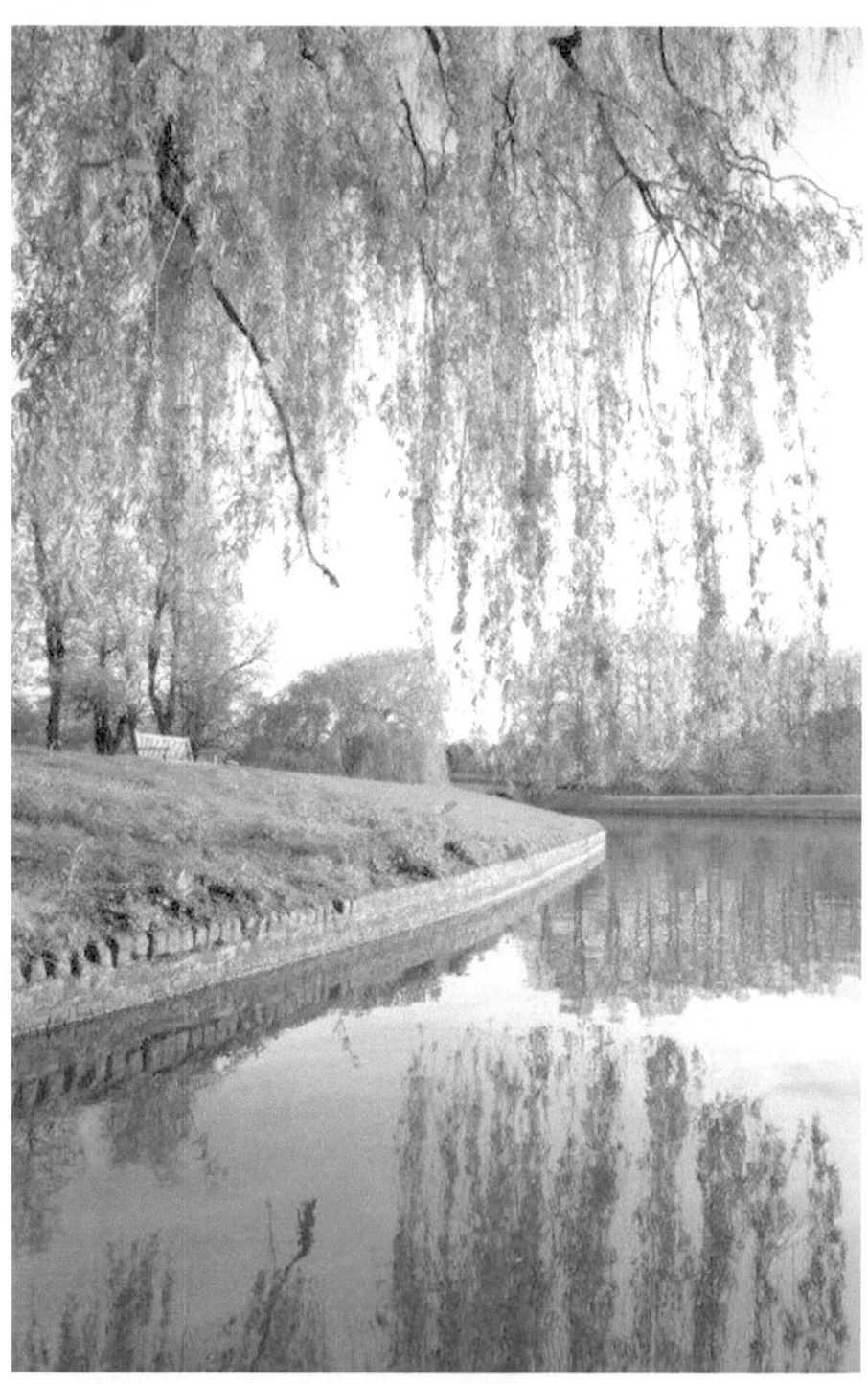

HYPERTENSION DIARY AND LOG

BLOOD PRESSURE LOG

Date / Day	Time	AM	PM	SYSTOLIC	DIASTOLIC	Pulse Rate

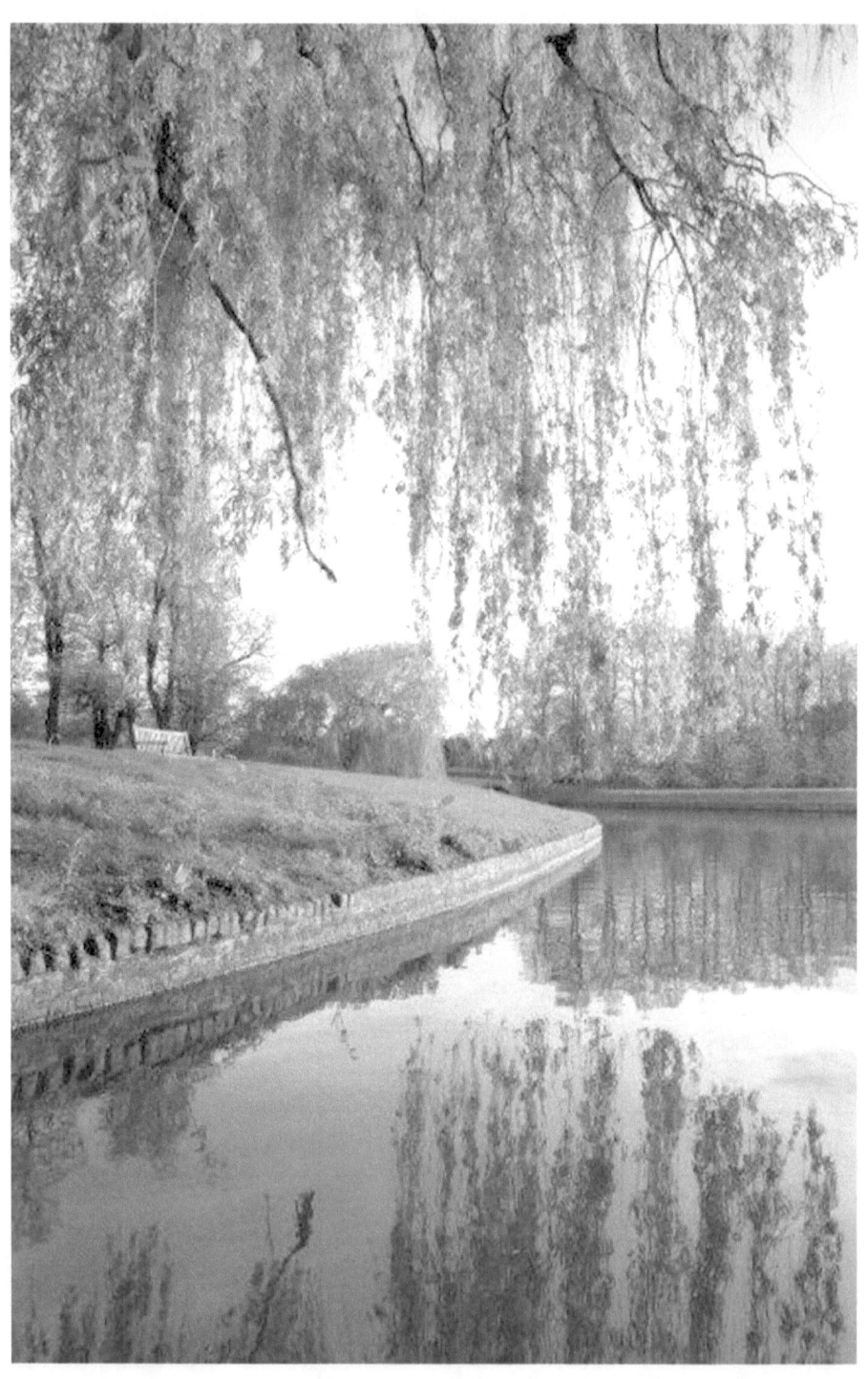

HYPERTENSION DIARY AND LOG

BLOOD PRESSURE LOG

Date / Day	Time	AM	PM	SYSTOLIC	DIASTOLIC	Pulse Rate

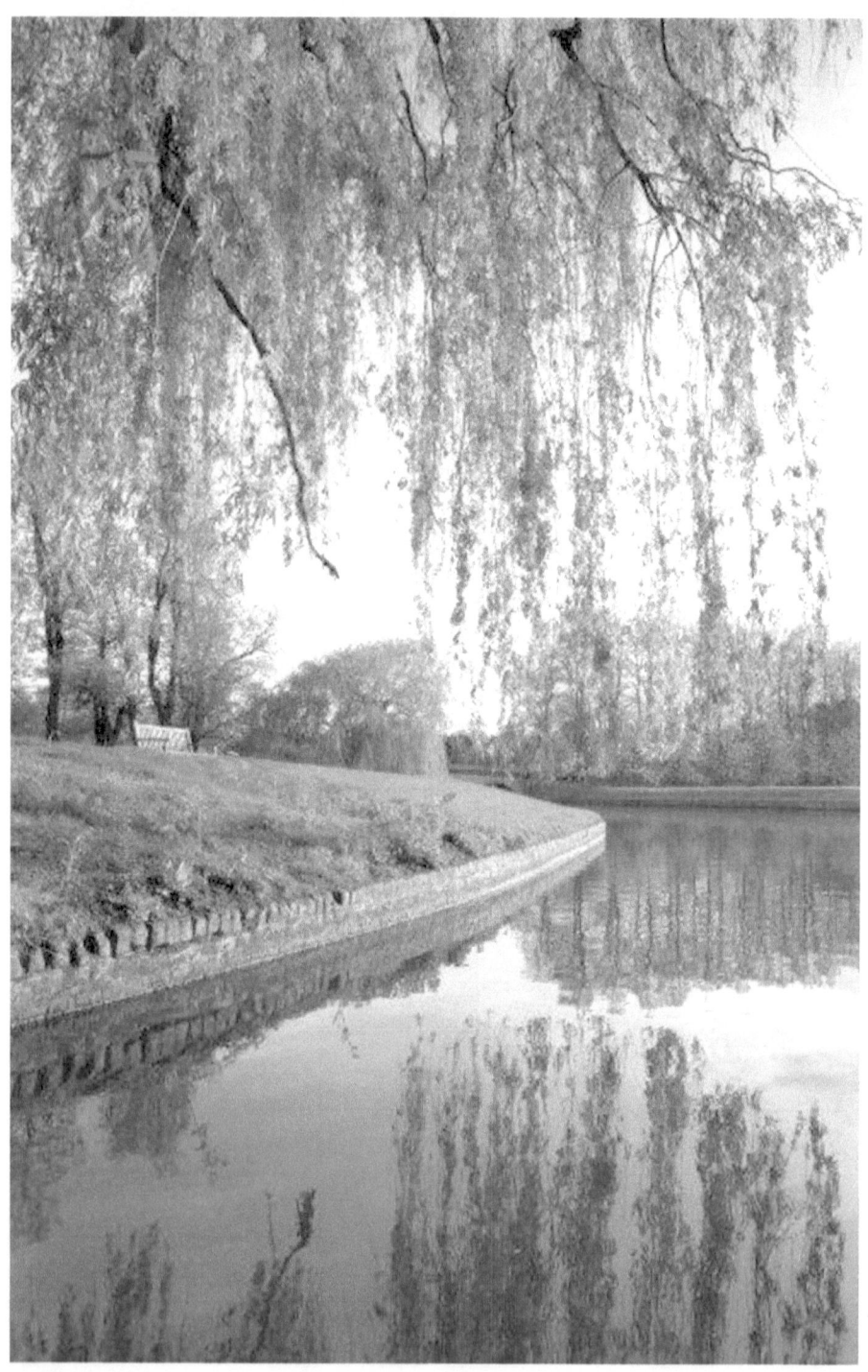

HYPERTENSION DIARY AND LOG

BLOOD PRESSURE LOG

Date / Day	Time	AM	PM	SYSTOLIC	DIASTOLIC	Pulse Rate

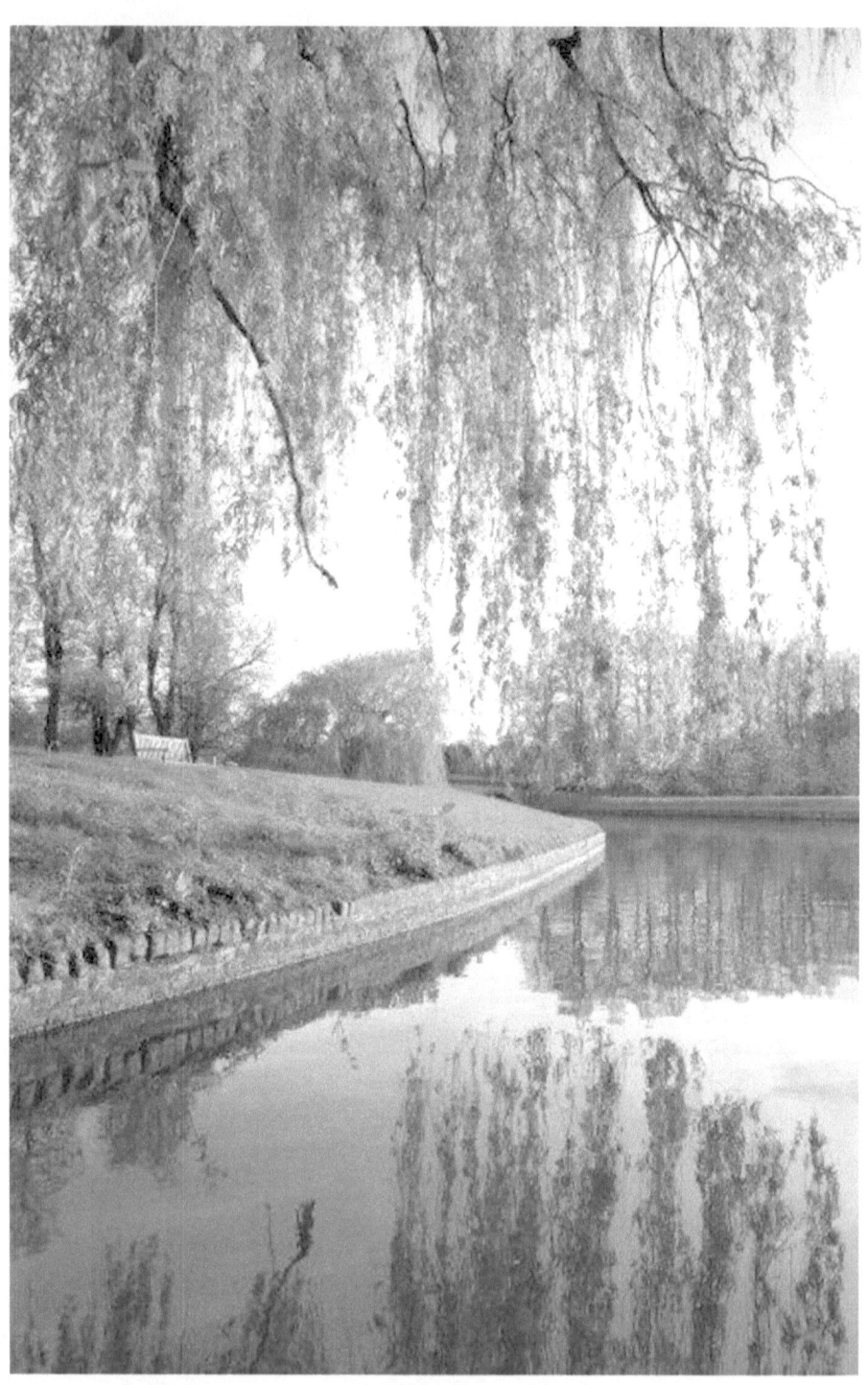

HYPERTENSION DIARY AND LOG

BLOOD PRESSURE LOG

Date / Day	Time	AM	PM	SYSTOLIC	DIASTOLIC	Pulse Rate

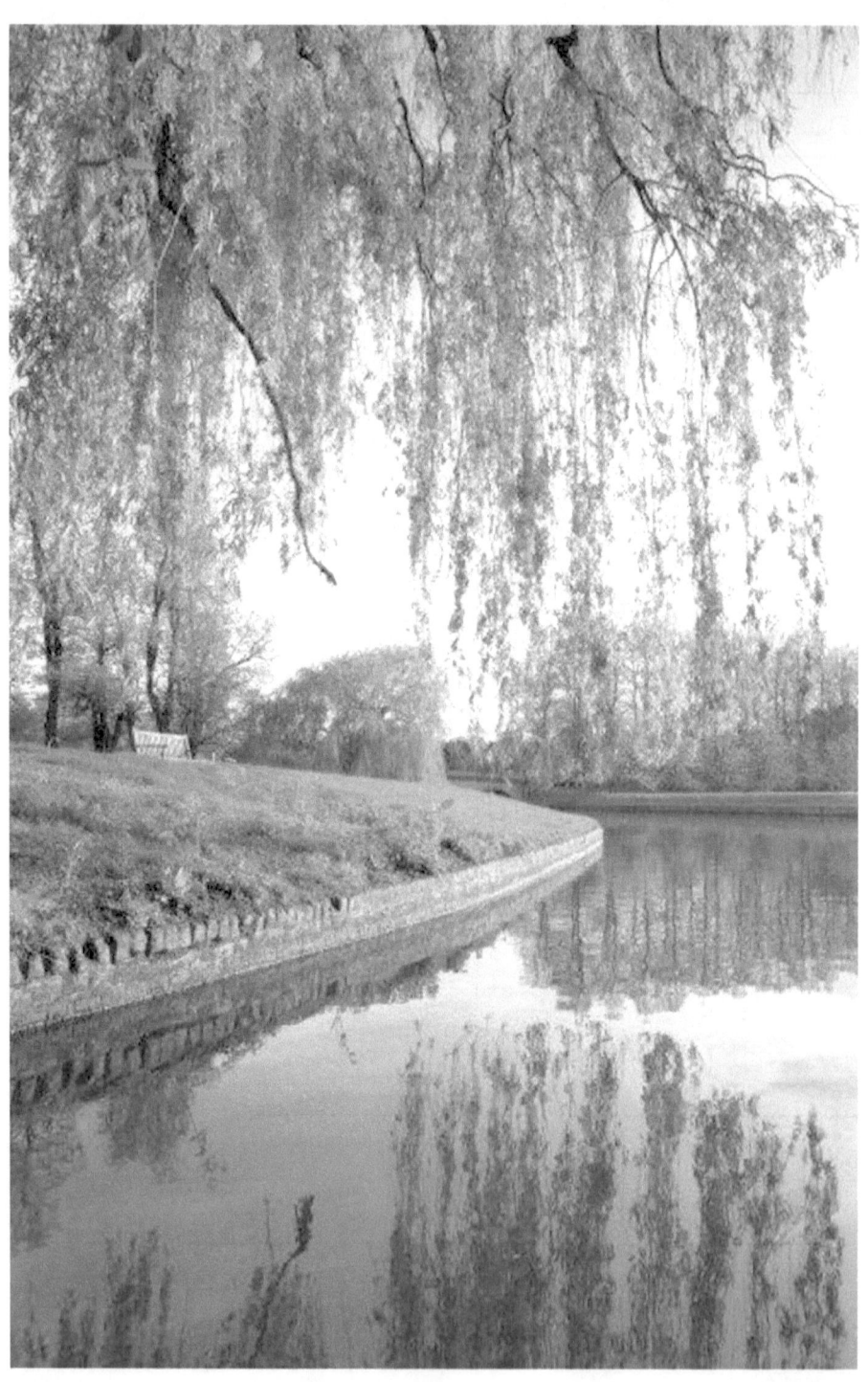

BLOOD PRESSURE LOG

Date / Day	Time	AM	PM	SYSTOLIC	DIASTOLIC	Pulse Rate

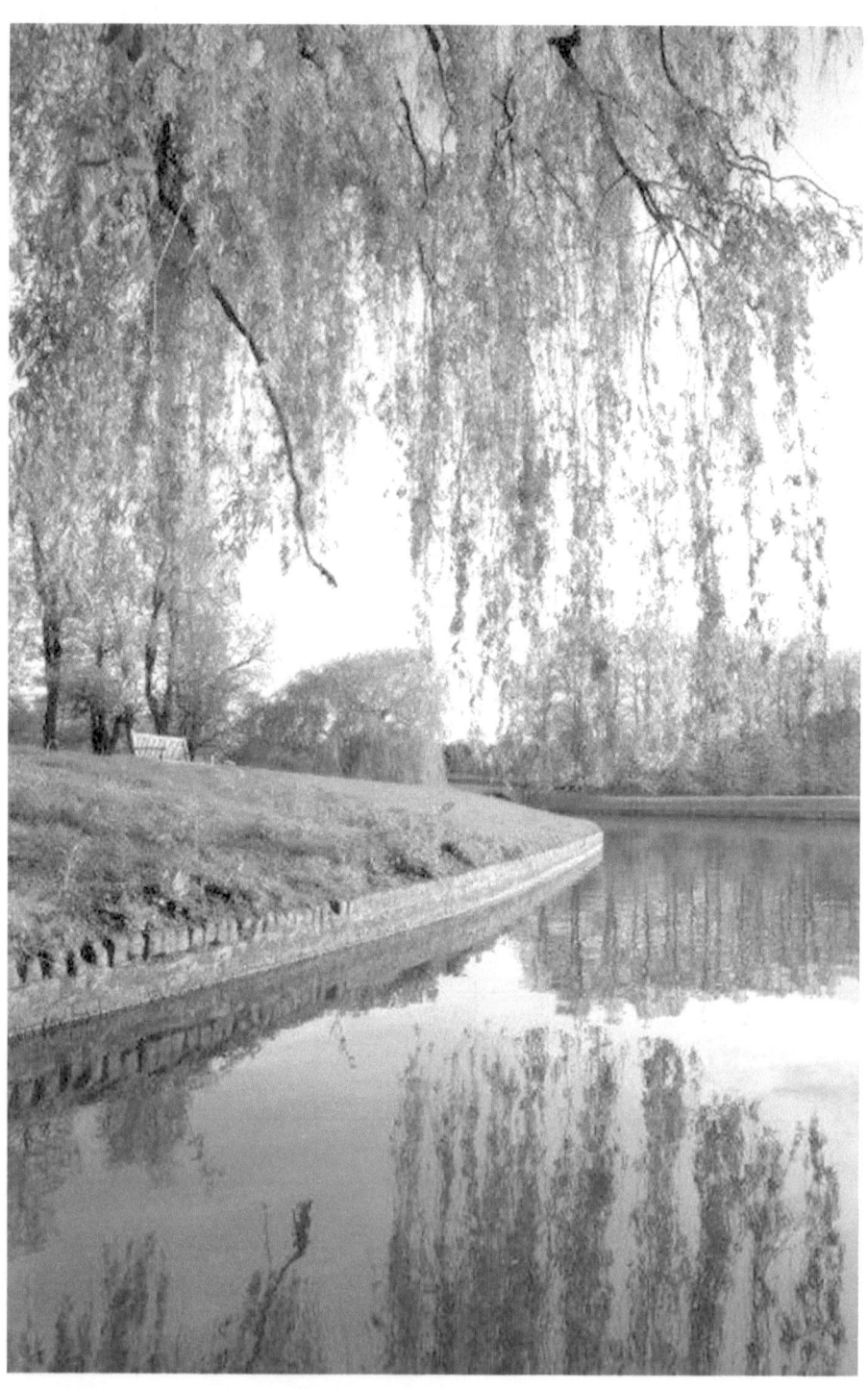

HYPERTENSION DIARY AND LOG

BLOOD PRESSURE LOG

Date / Day	Time	AM	PM	SYSTOLIC	DIASTOLIC	Pulse Rate

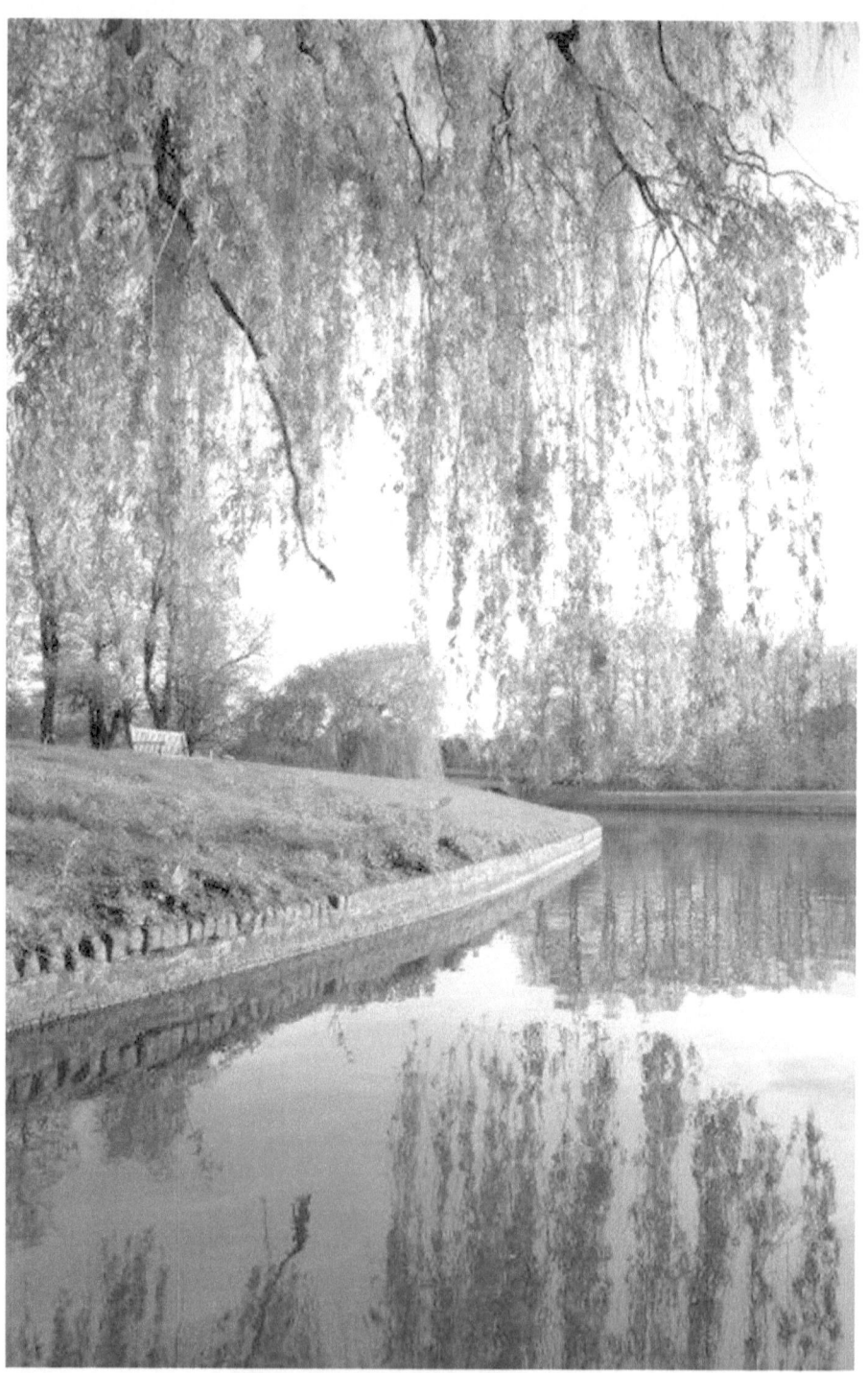

HYPERTENSION DIARY AND LOG

BLOOD PRESSURE LOG

Date / Day	Time	AM	PM	SYSTOLIC	DIASTOLIC	Pulse Rate

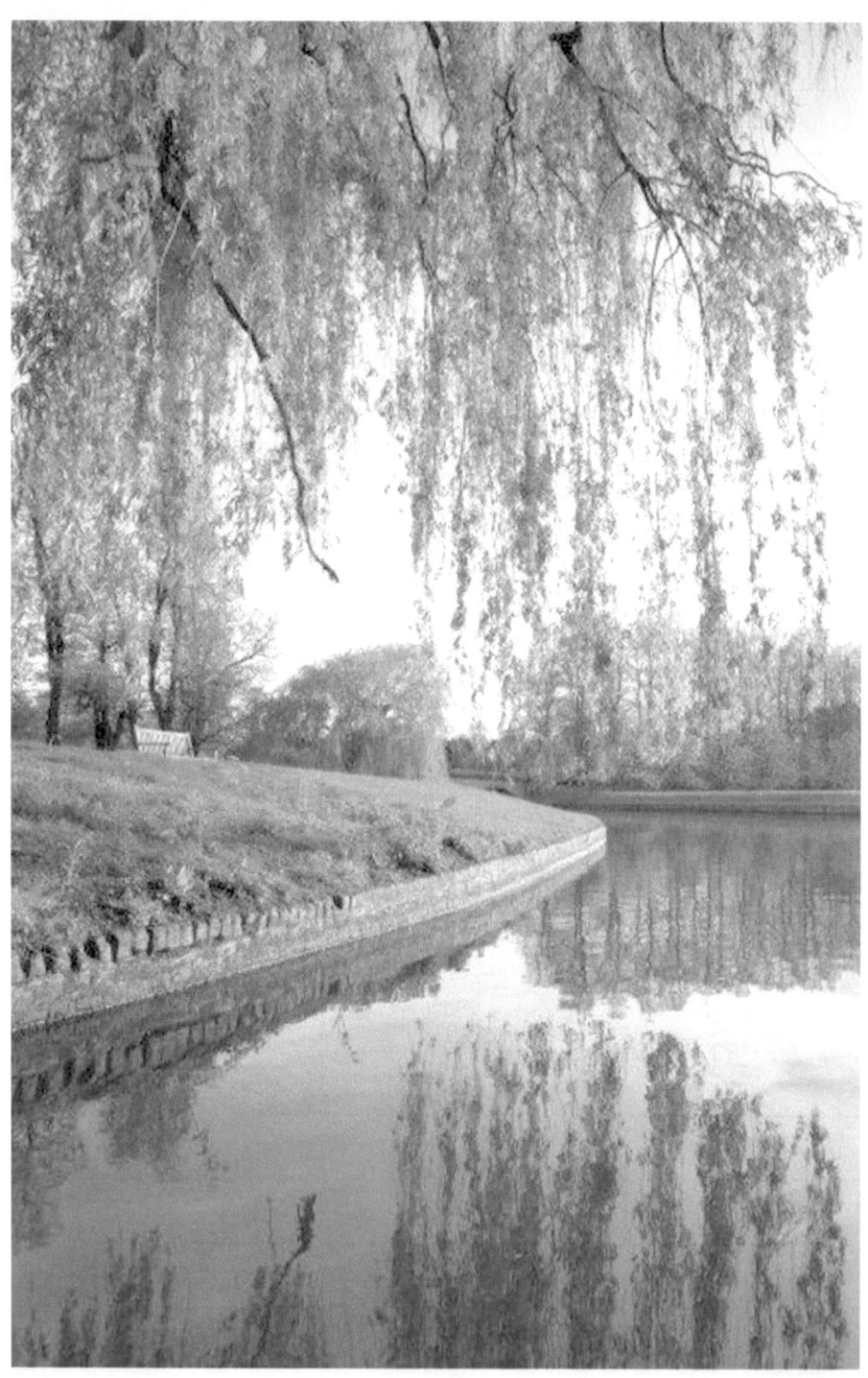

BLOOD PRESSURE LOG

Date / Day	Time	AM	PM	SYSTOLIC	DIASTOLIC	Pulse Rate

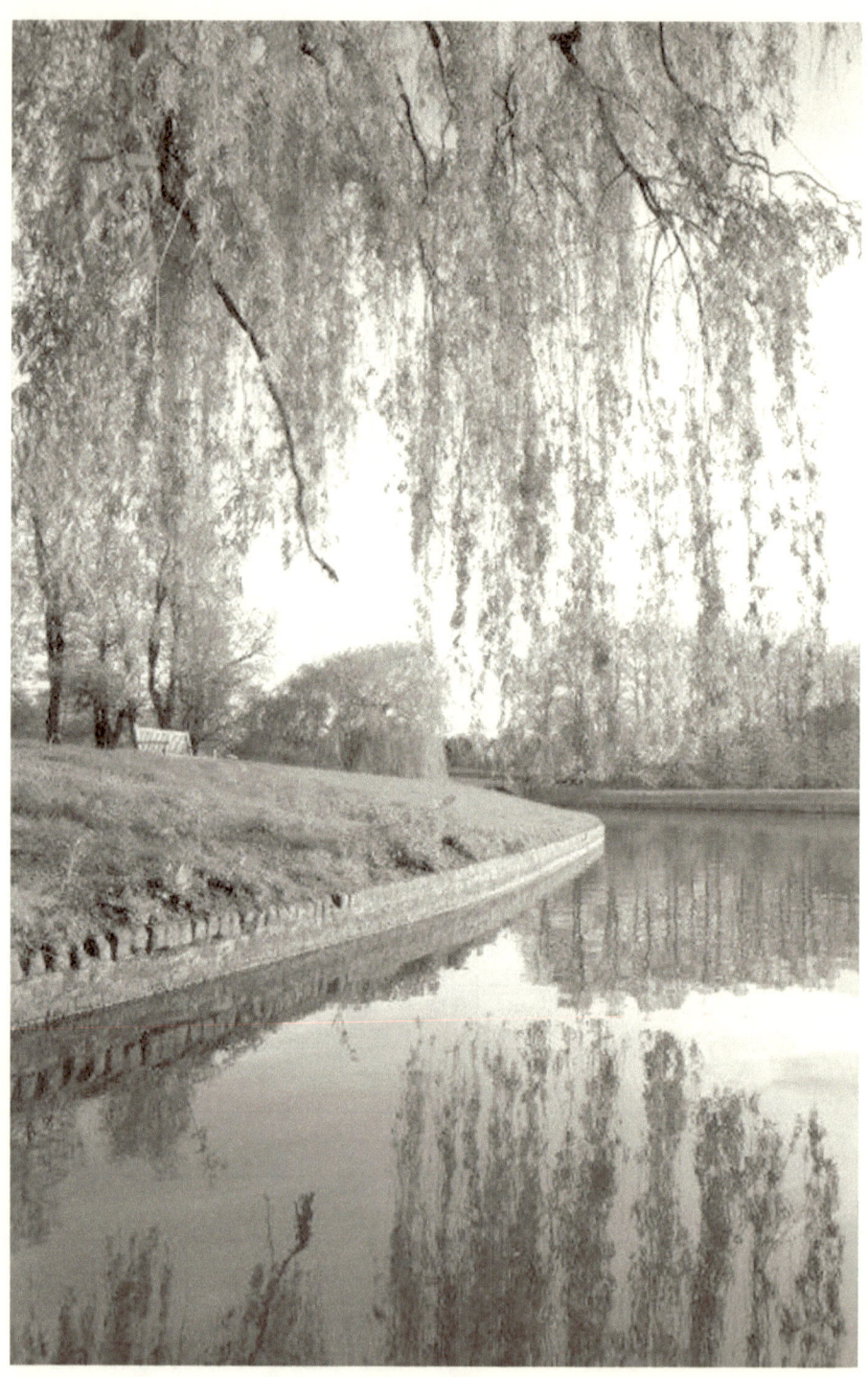

HYPERTENSION DIARY AND LOG

BLOOD PRESSURE LOG

Date / Day	Time	AM	PM	SYSTOLIC	DIASTOLIC	Pulse Rate

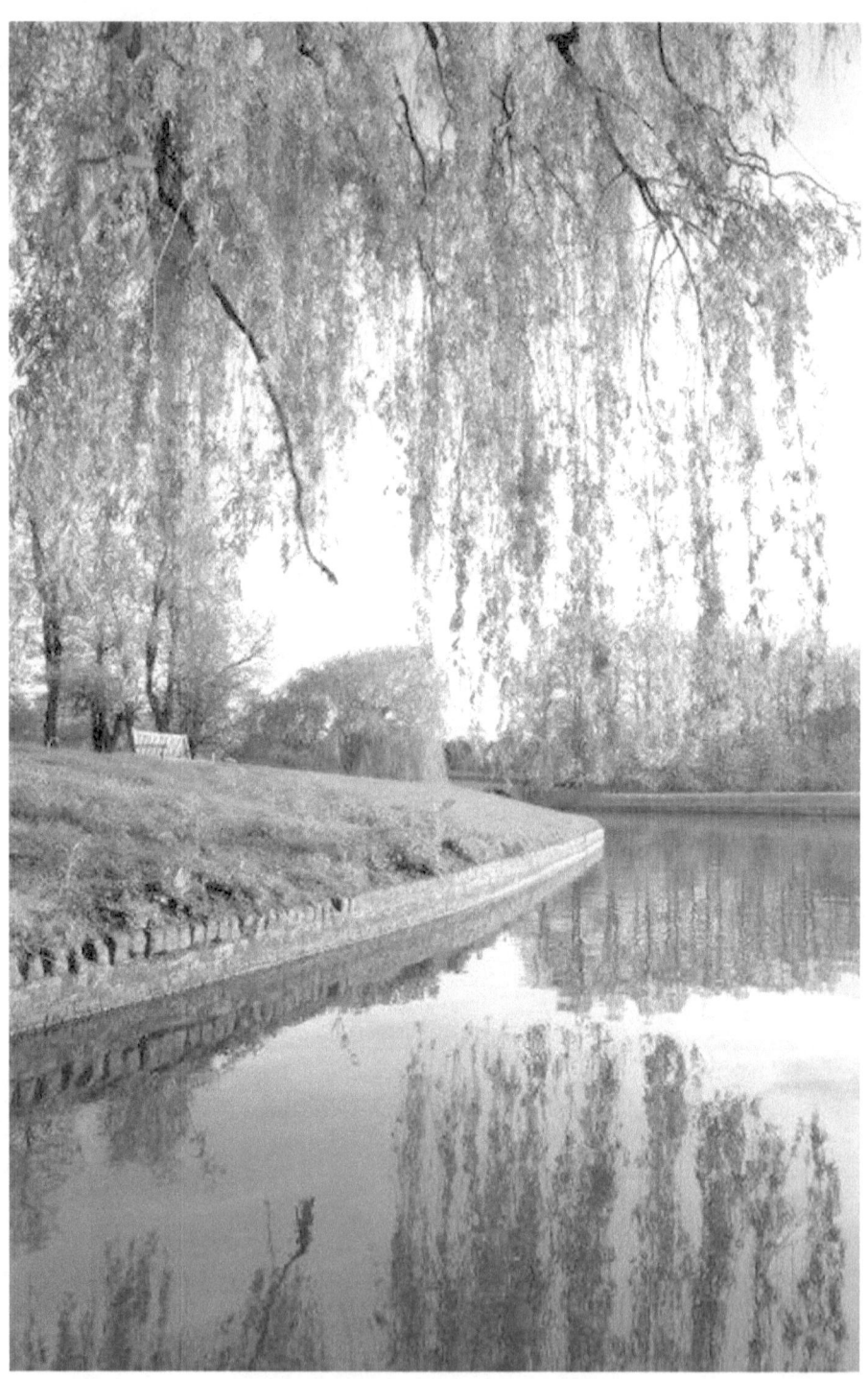

BLOOD PRESSURE LOG

Date / Day	Time	AM	PM	SYSTOLIC	DIASTOLIC	Pulse Rate

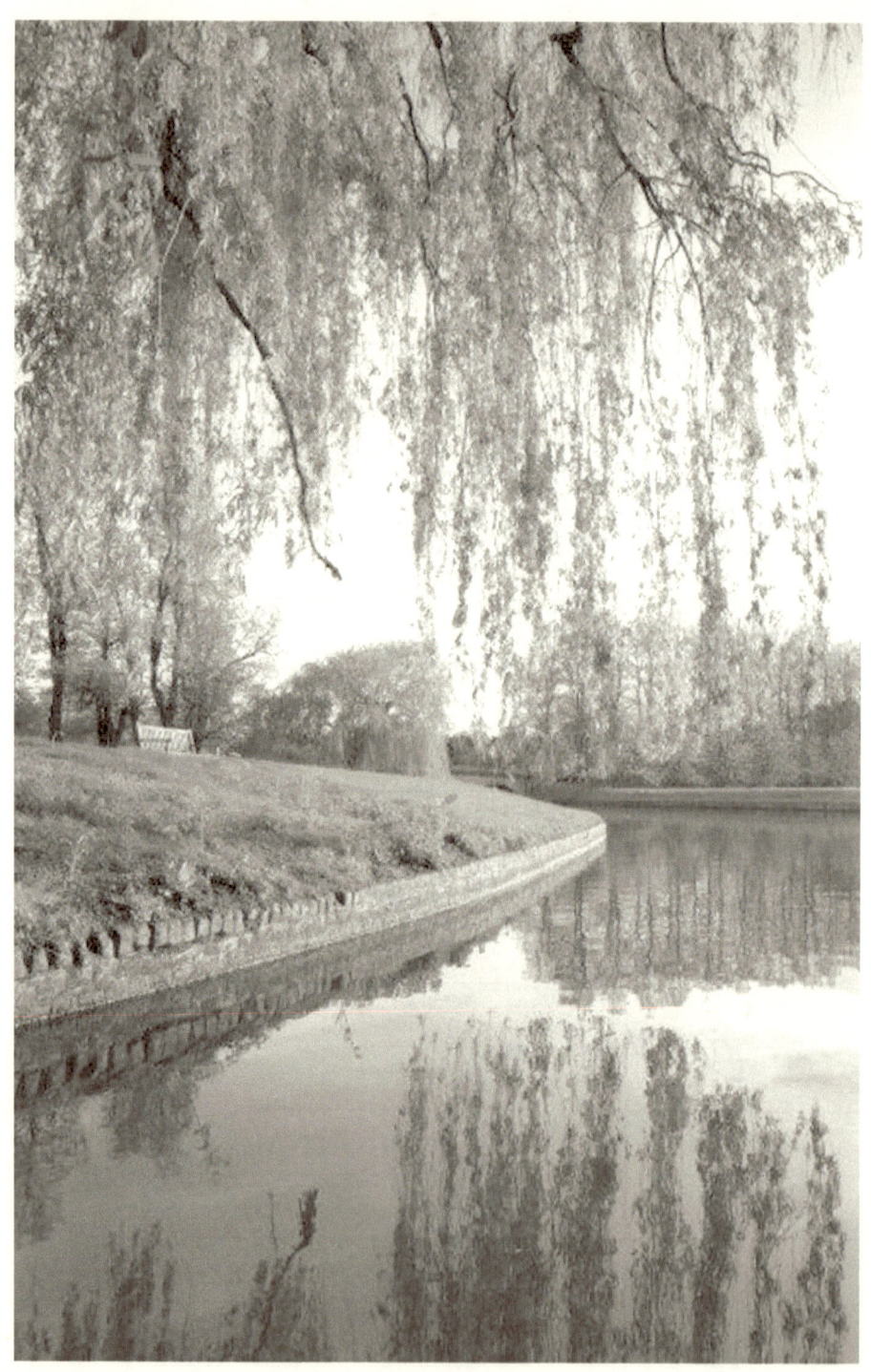

HYPERTENSION DIARY AND LOG

BLOOD PRESSURE LOG

Date / Day	Time	AM	PM	SYSTOLIC	DIASTOLIC	Pulse Rate

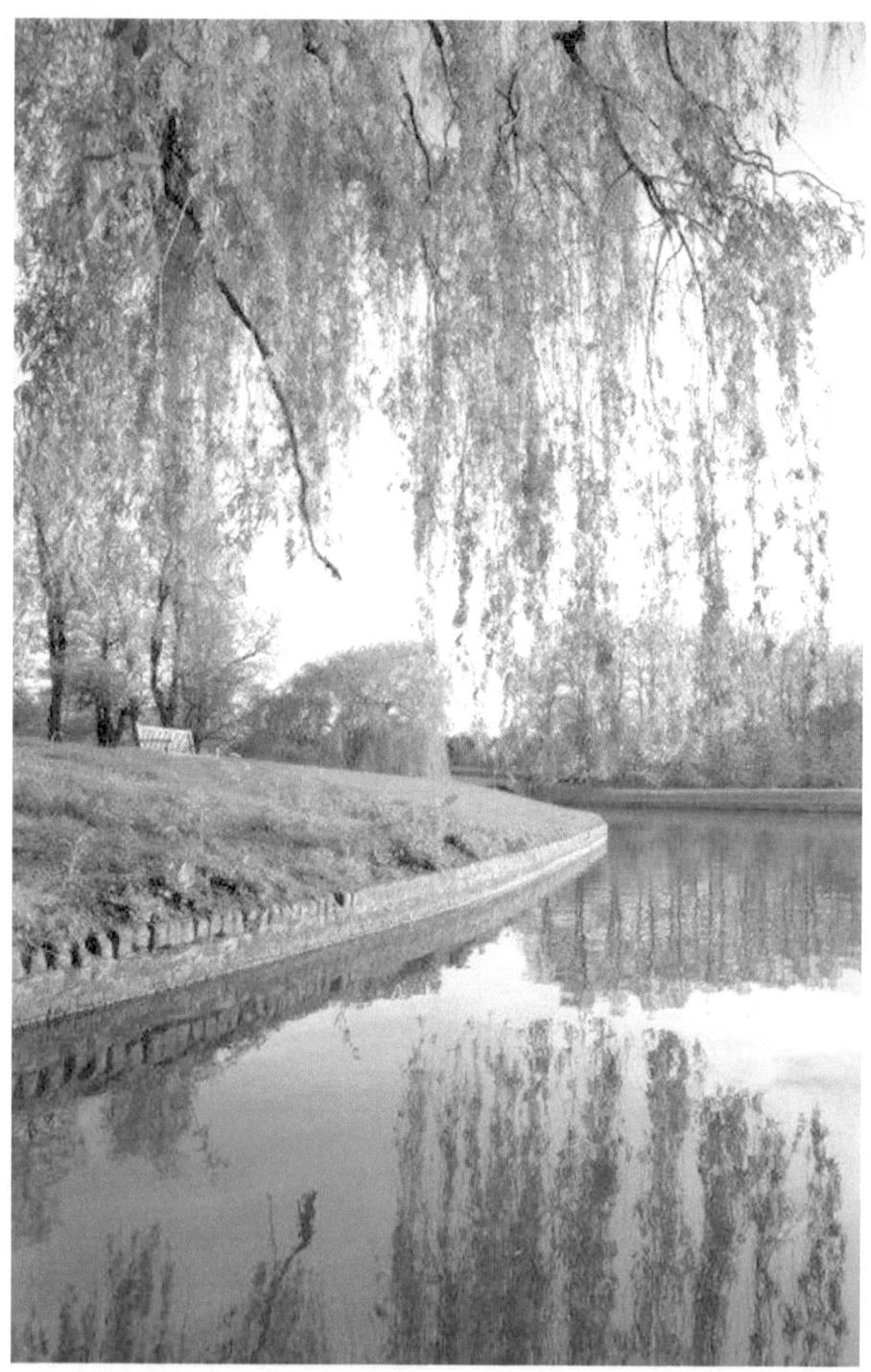

HYPERTENSION DIARY AND LOG

BLOOD PRESSURE LOG

Date / Day	Time	AM	PM	SYSTOLIC	DIASTOLIC	Pulse Rate

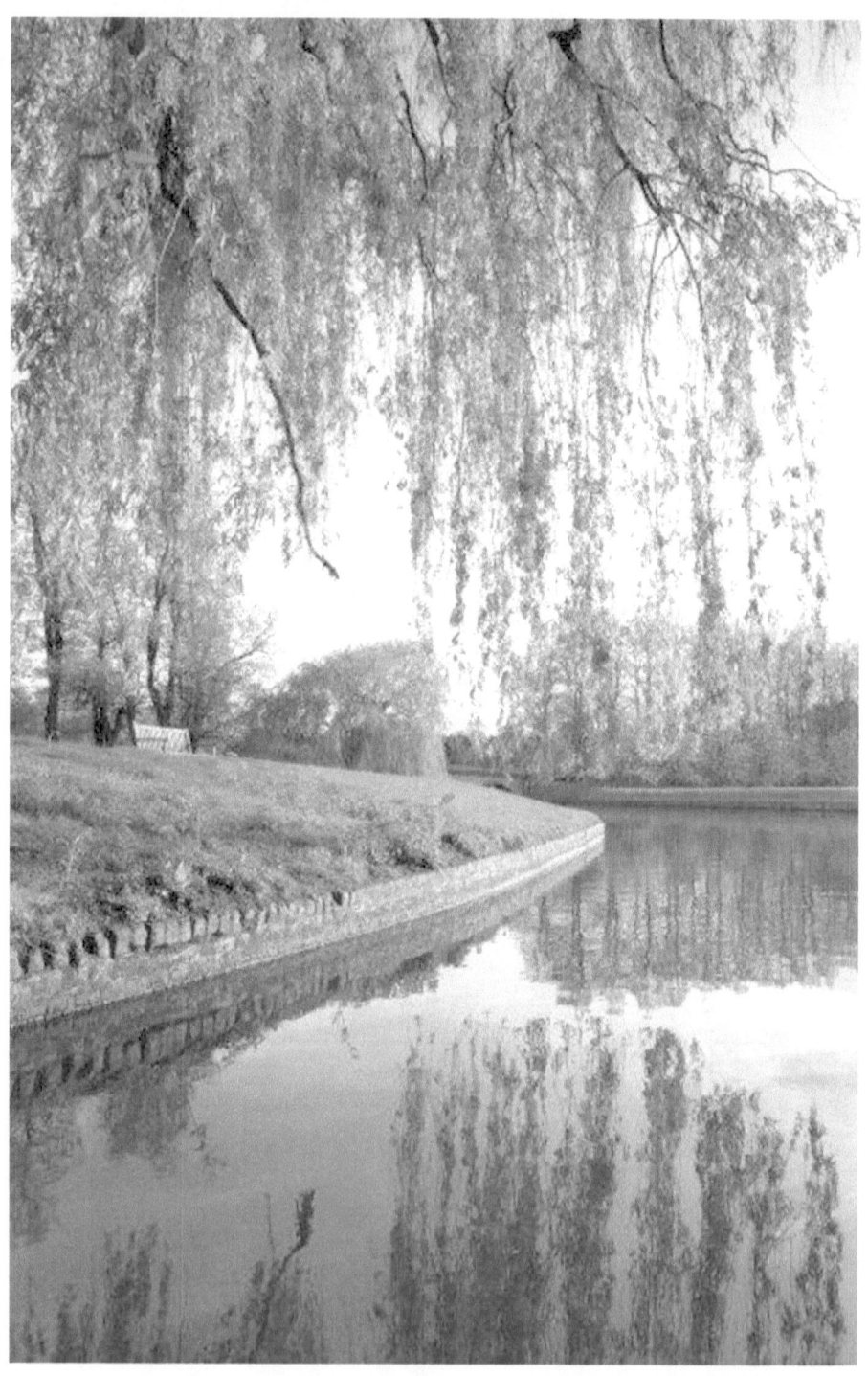

HYPERTENSION DIARY AND LOG

BLOOD PRESSURE LOG

Date / Day	Time	AM	PM	SYSTOLIC	DIASTOLIC	Pulse Rate

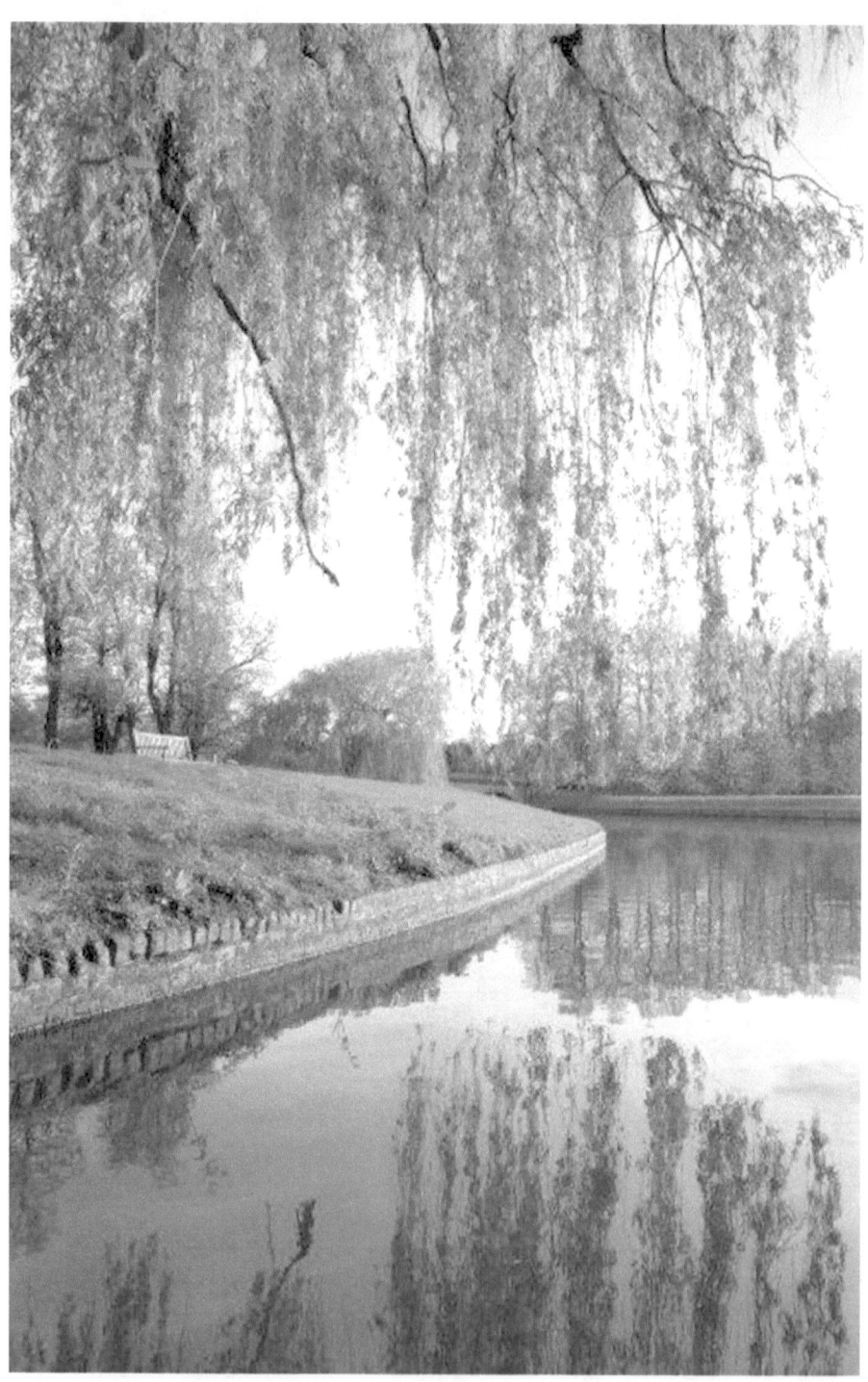

HYPERTENSION DIARY AND LOG

BLOOD PRESSURE LOG

Date / Day	Time	AM	PM	SYSTOLIC	DIASTOLIC	Pulse Rate

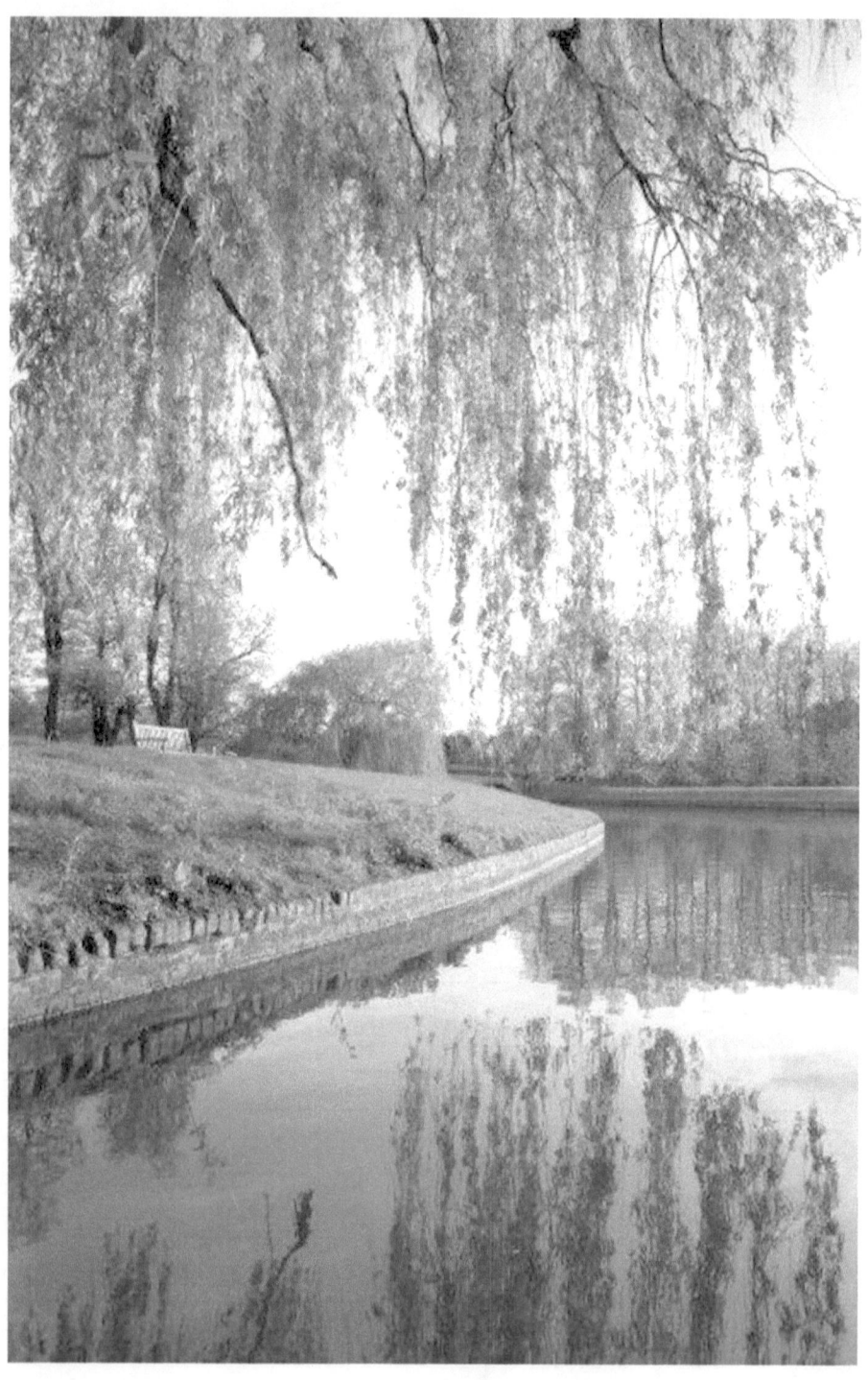

HYPERTENSION DIARY AND LOG

BLOOD PRESSURE LOG

Date / Day	Time	AM	PM	SYSTOLIC	DIASTOLIC	Pulse Rate

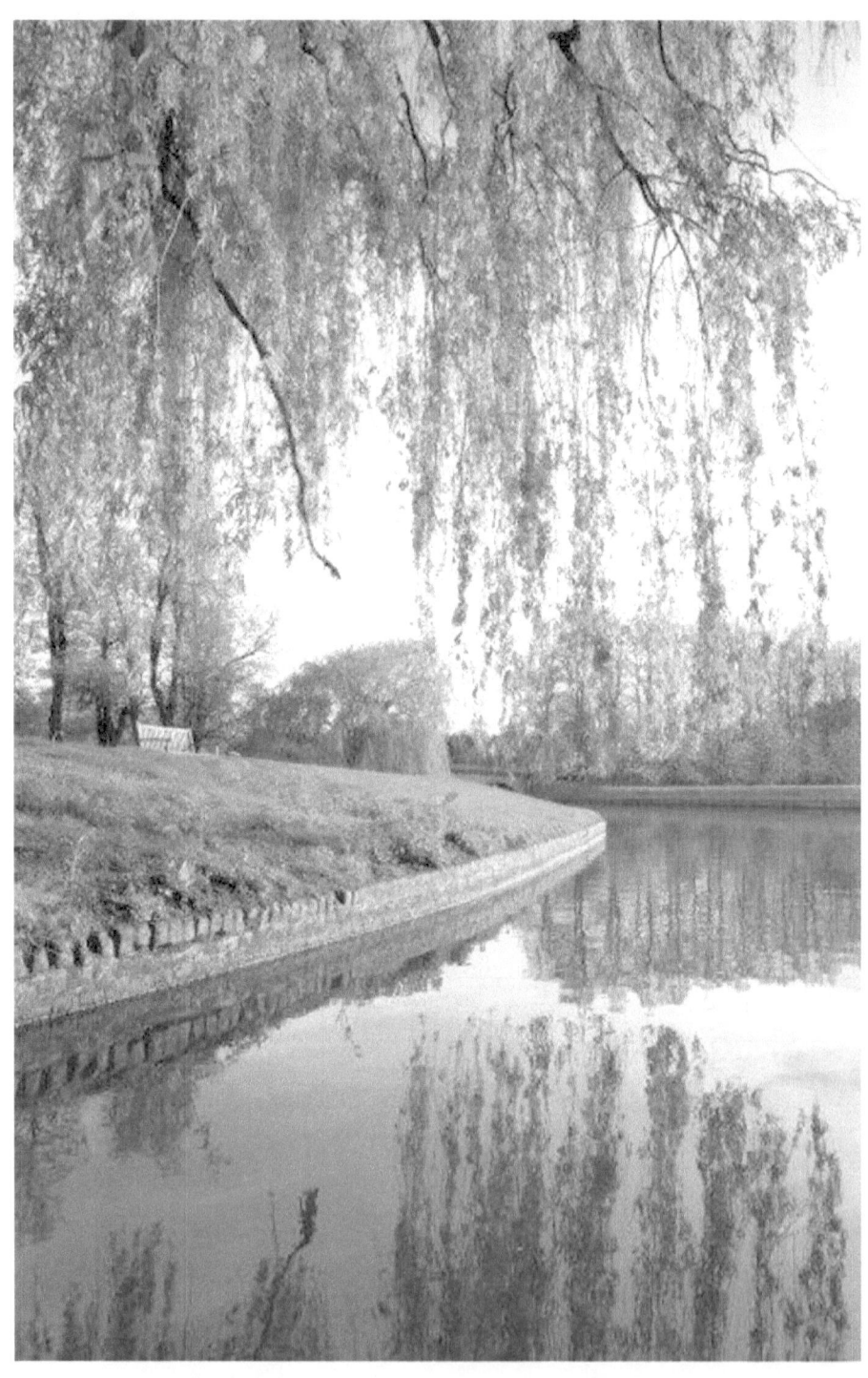

HYPERTENSION DIARY AND LOG

BLOOD PRESSURE LOG

Date / Day	Time	AM	PM	SYSTOLIC	DIASTOLIC	Pulse Rate

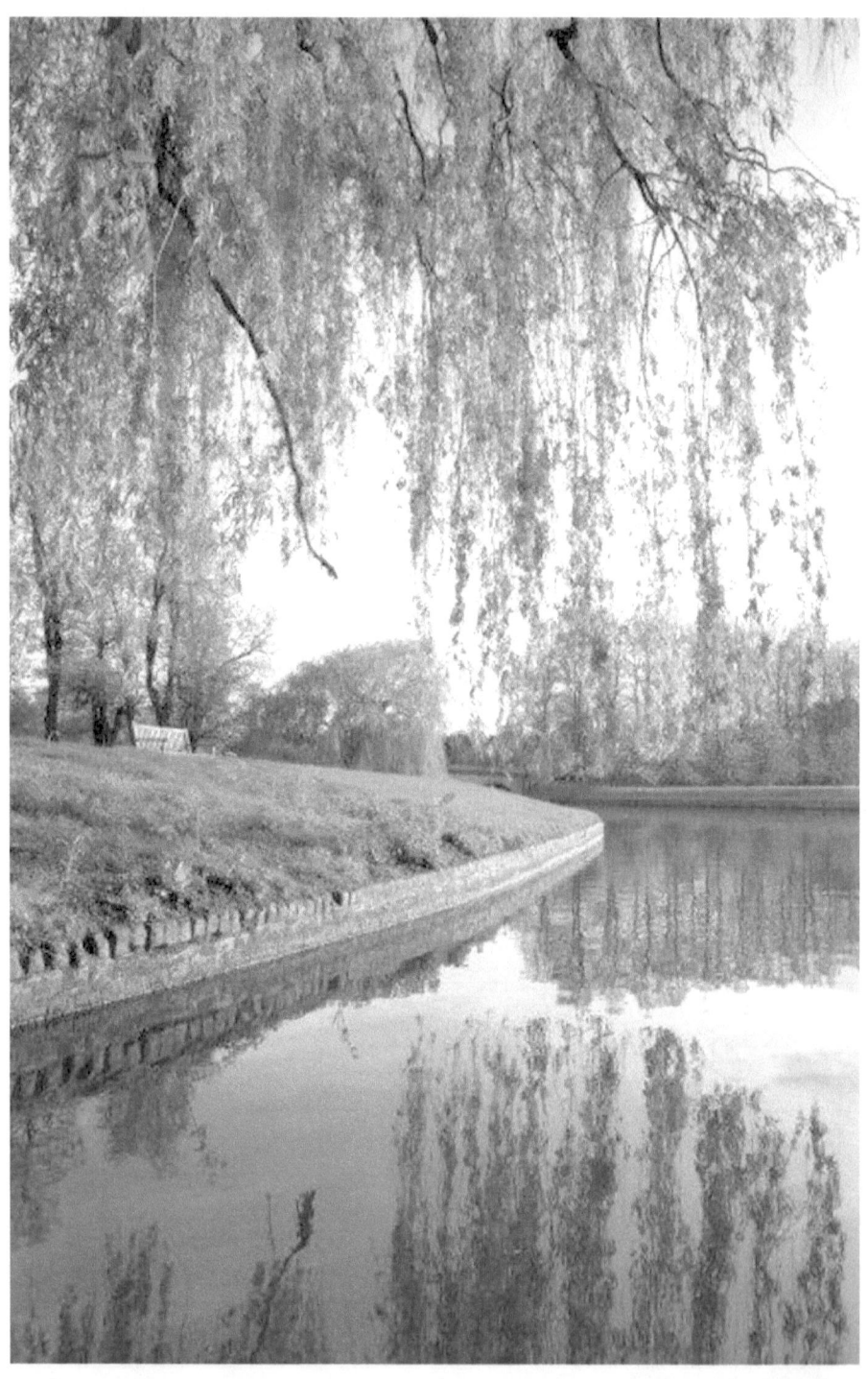

HYPERTENSION DIARY AND LOG

BLOOD PRESSURE LOG

Date / Day	Time	AM	PM	SYSTOLIC	DIASTOLIC	Pulse Rate

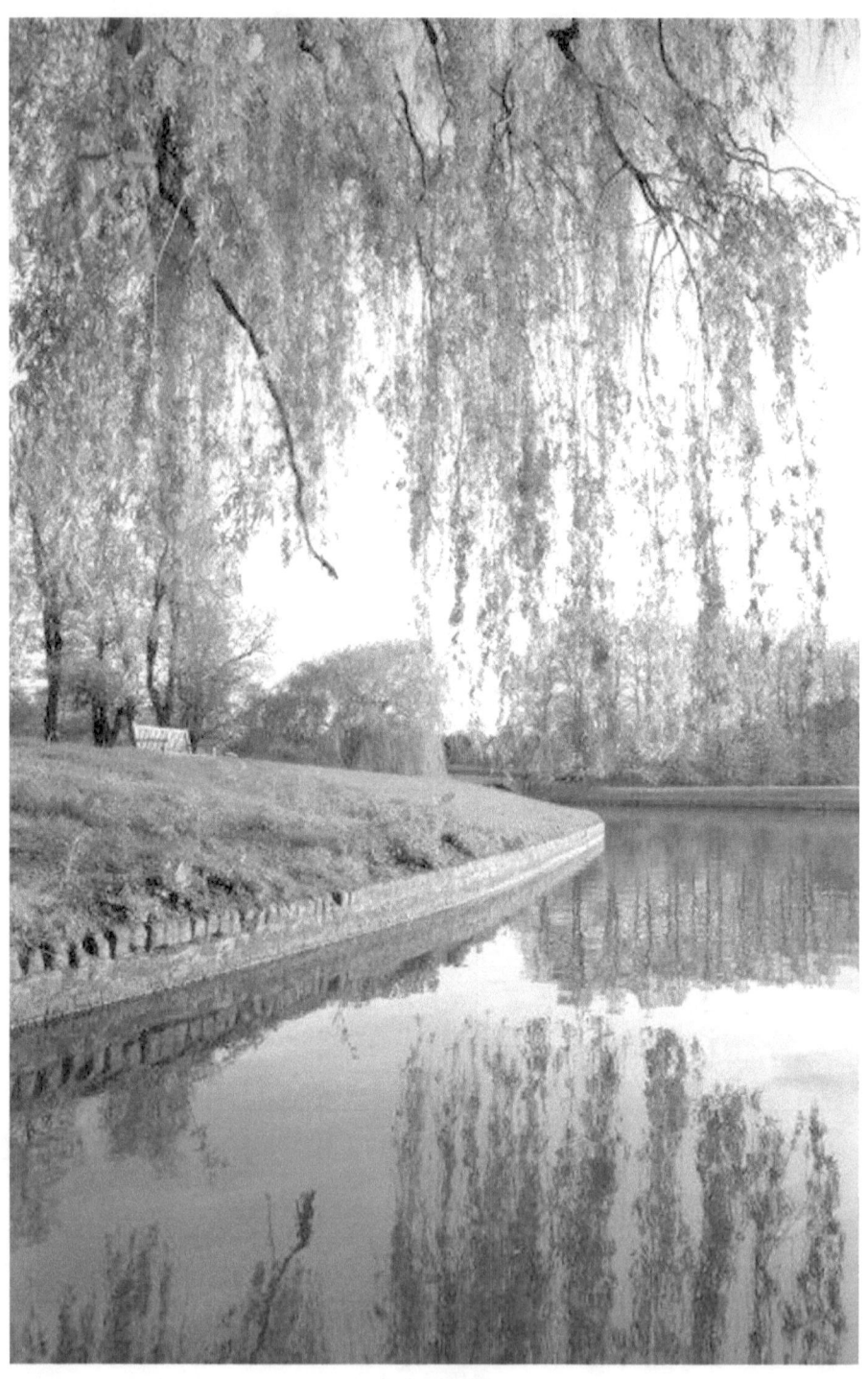

HYPERTENSION DIARY AND LOG

BLOOD PRESSURE LOG

Date / Day	Time	AM	PM	SYSTOLIC	DIASTOLIC	Pulse Rate

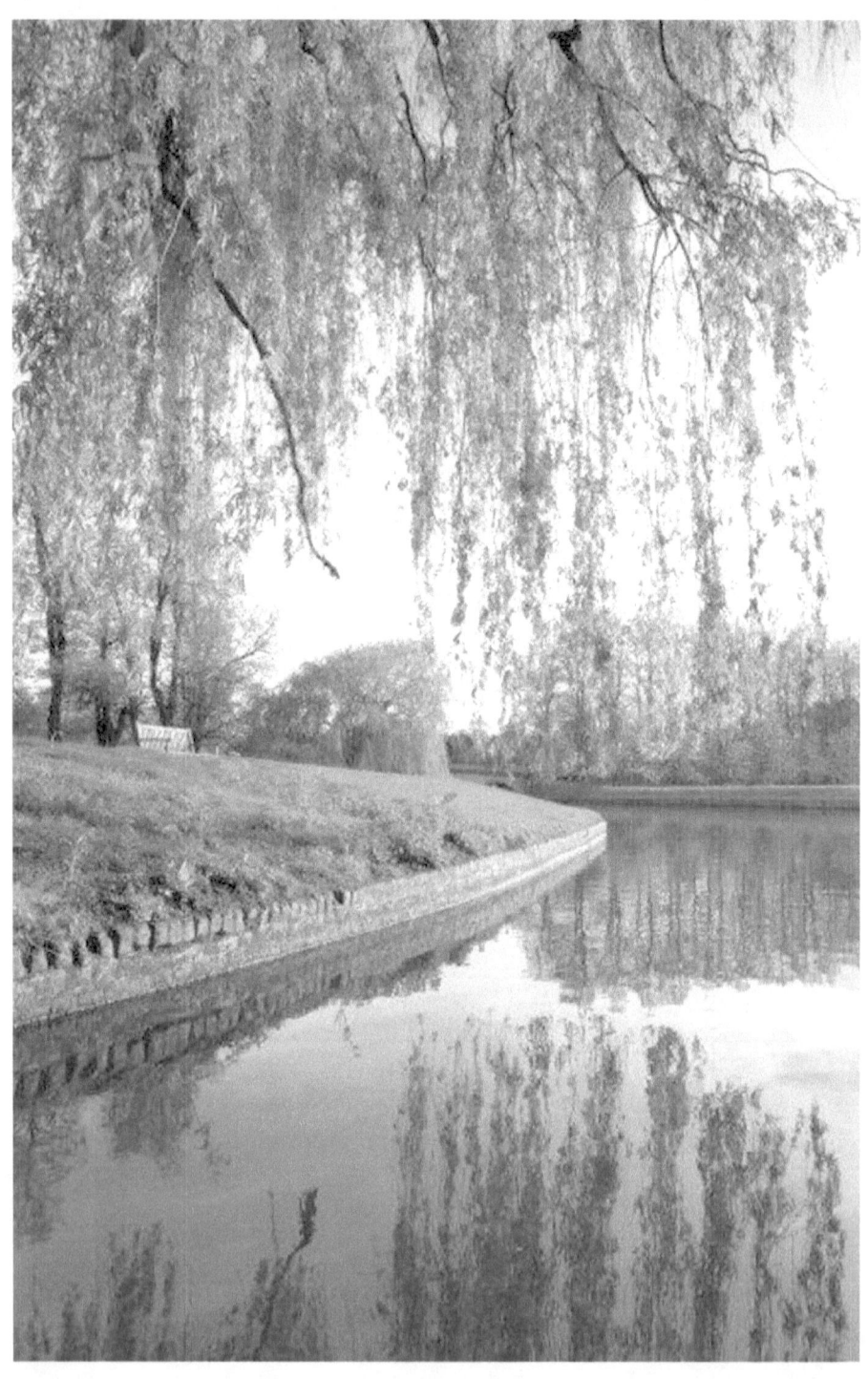

HYPERTENSION DIARY AND LOG

BLOOD PRESSURE LOG

Date / Day	Time	AM	PM	SYSTOLIC	DIASTOLIC	Pulse Rate

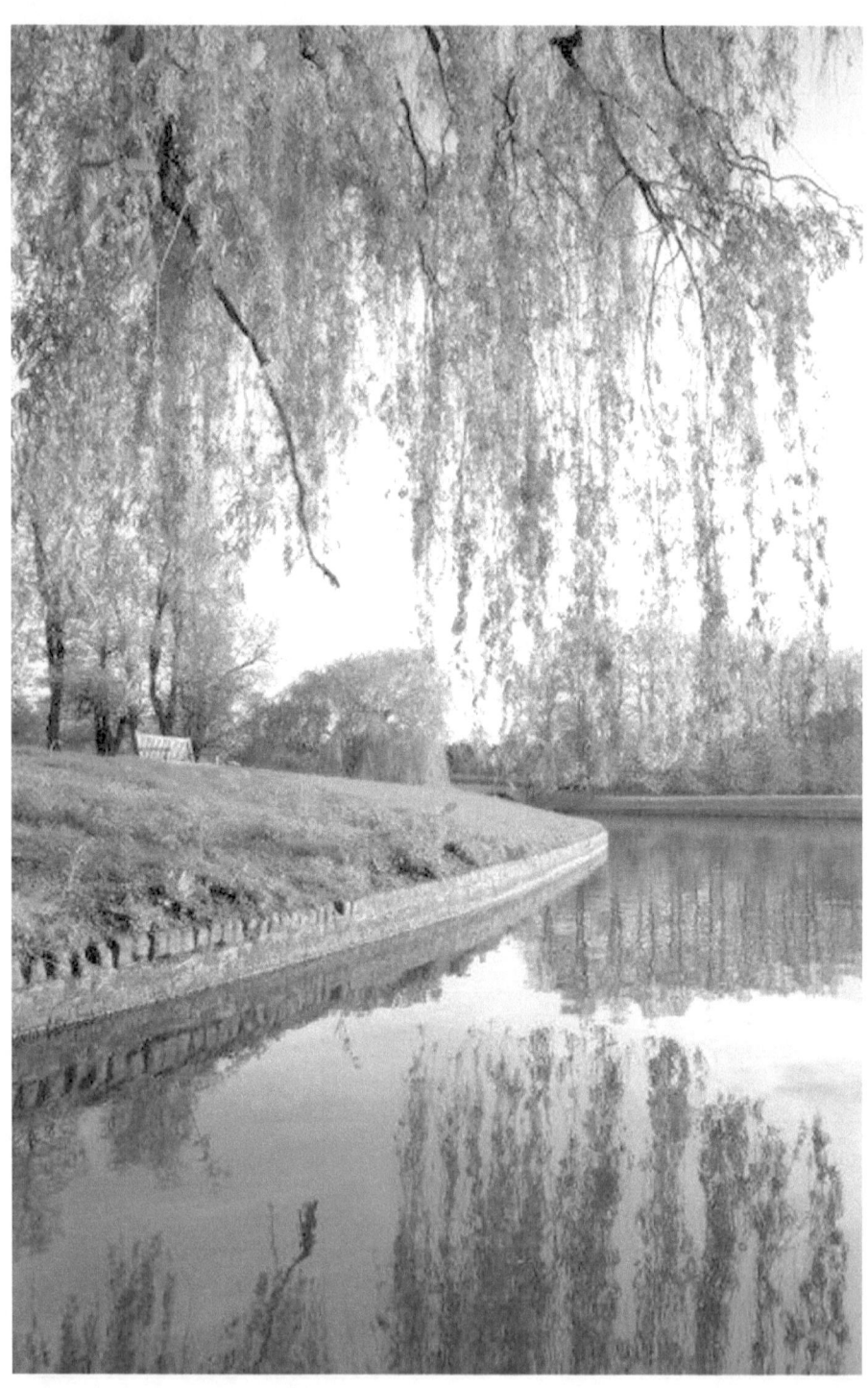

HYPERTENSION DIARY AND LOG

BLOOD PRESSURE LOG

Date / Day	Time	AM	PM	SYSTOLIC	DIASTOLIC	Pulse Rate

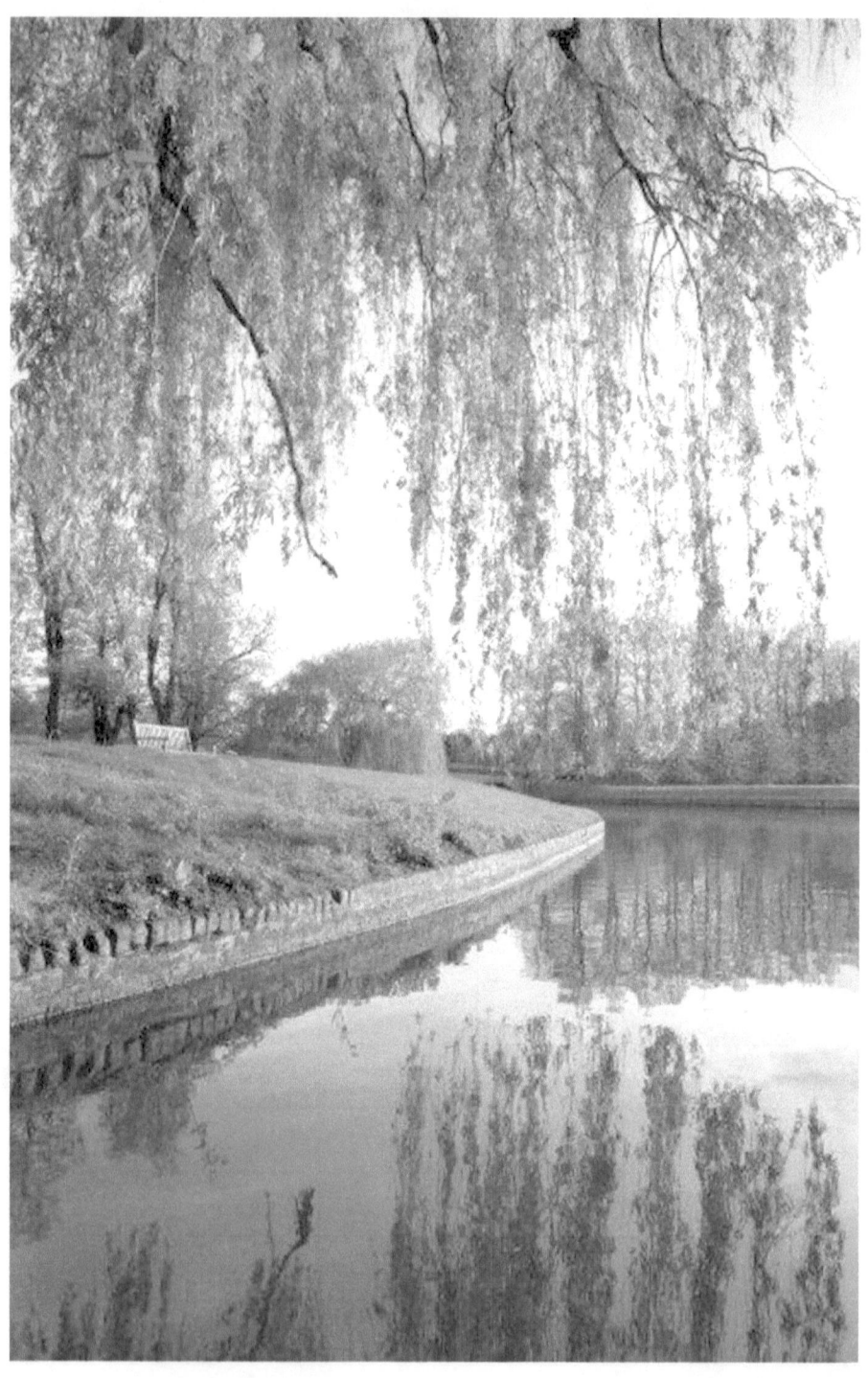

HYPERTENSION DIARY AND LOG

BLOOD PRESSURE LOG

Date / Day	Time	AM	PM	SYSTOLIC	DIASTOLIC	Pulse Rate

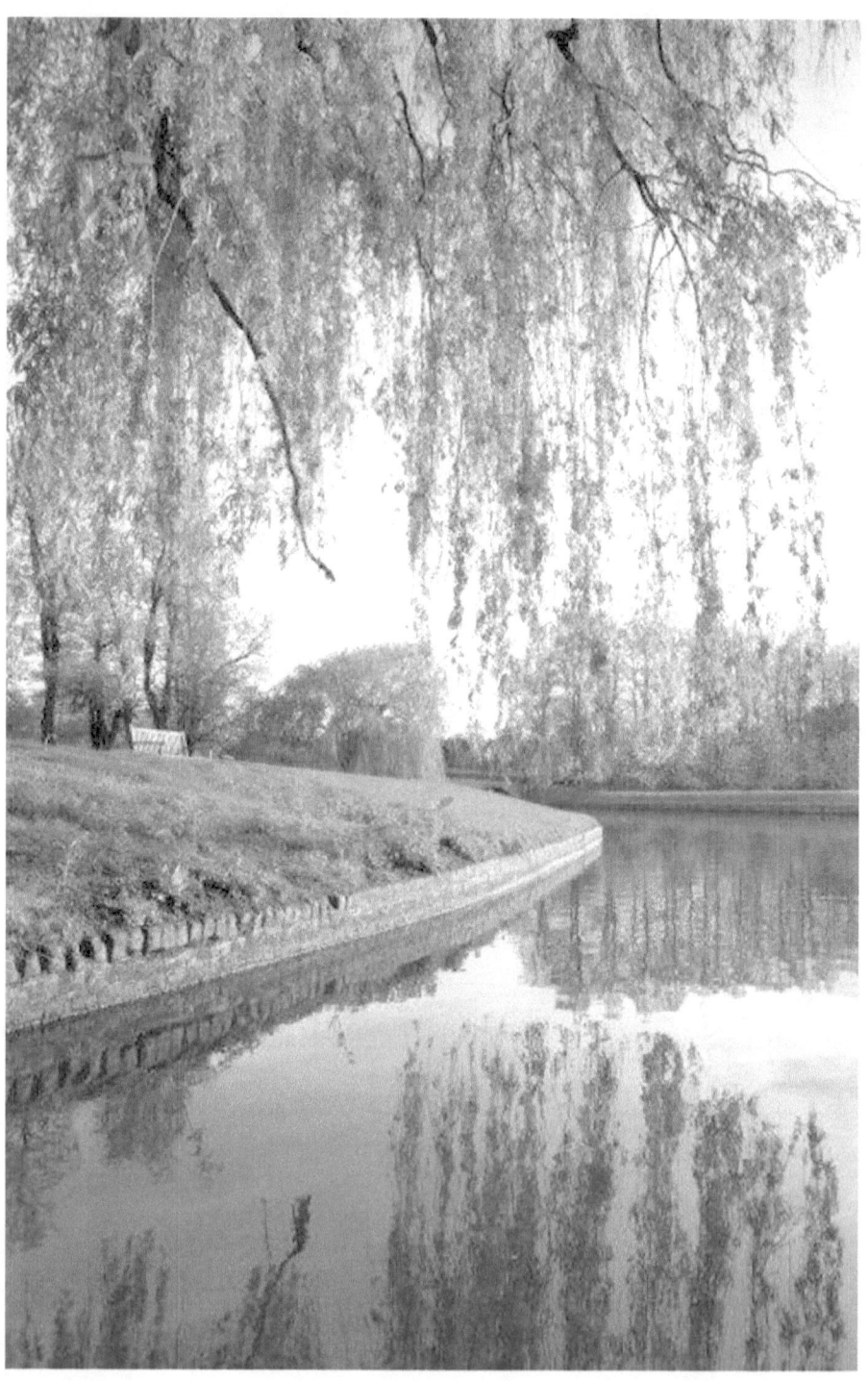

HYPERTENSION DIARY AND LOG

BLOOD PRESSURE LOG

Date / Day	Time	AM	PM	SYSTOLIC	DIASTOLIC	Pulse Rate

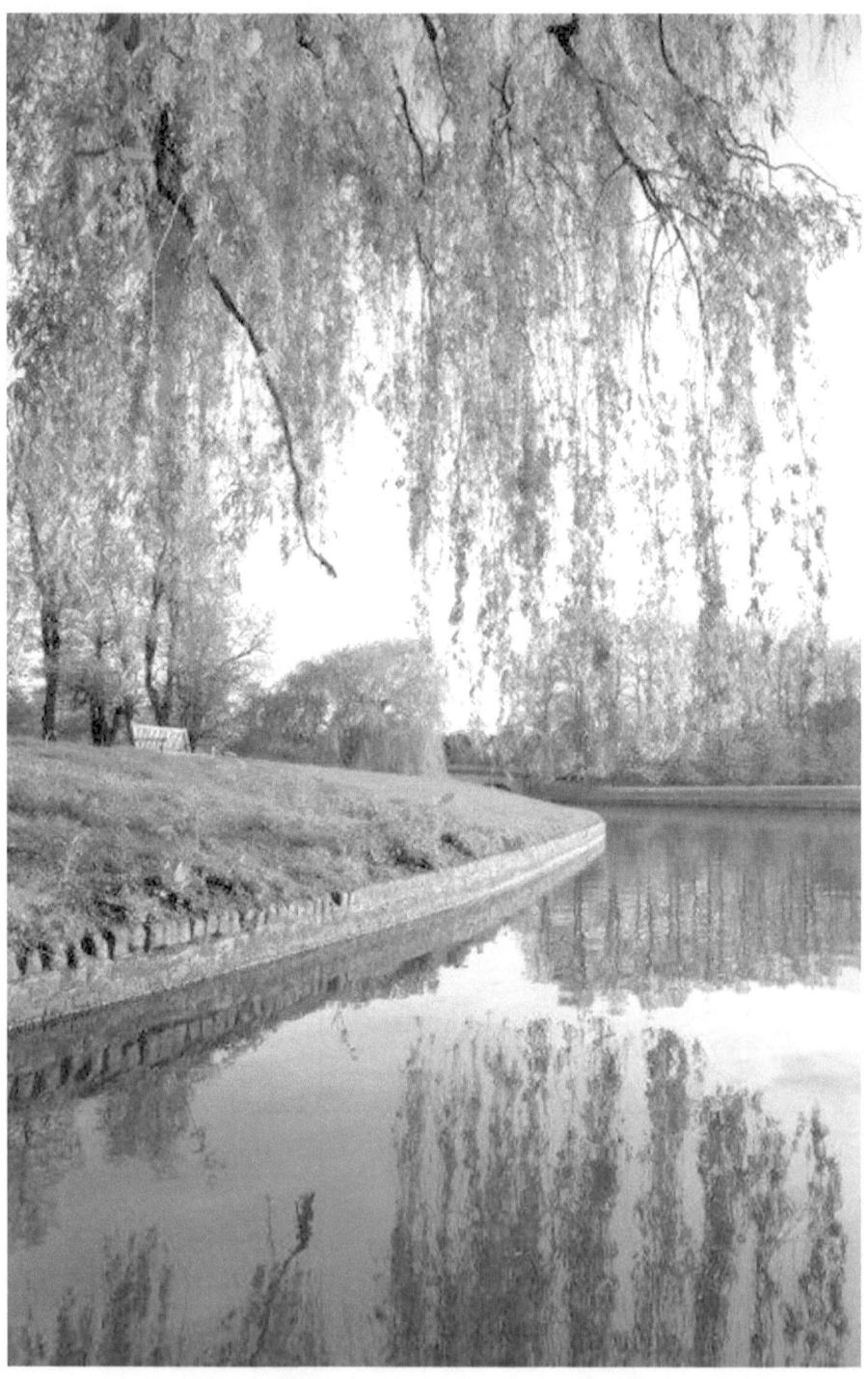

BLOOD PRESSURE LOG

Date / Day	Time	AM	PM	SYSTOLIC	DIASTOLIC	Pulse Rate

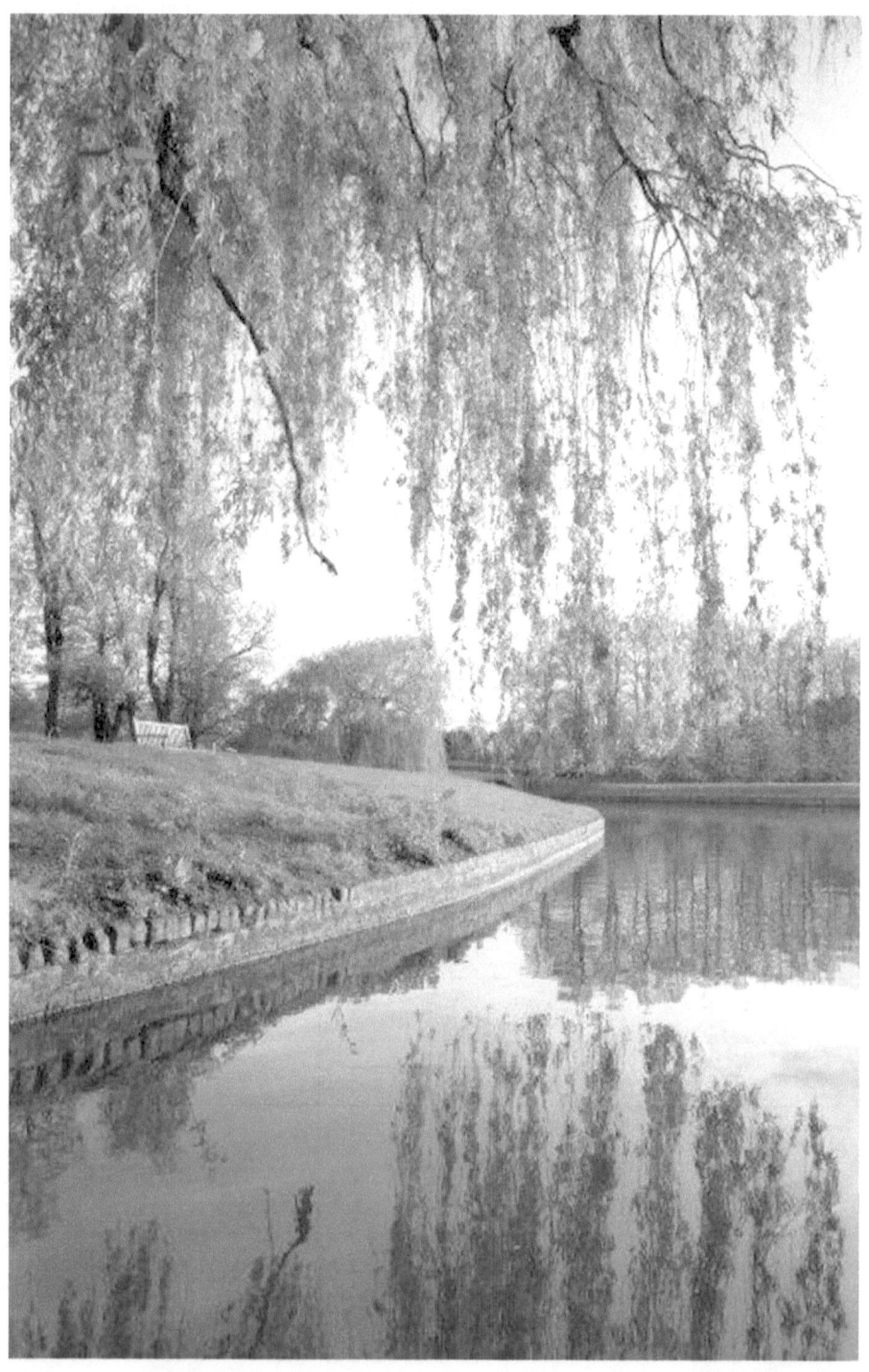

HYPERTENSION DIARY AND LOG

BLOOD PRESSURE LOG

Date / Day	Time	AM	PM	SYSTOLIC	DIASTOLIC	Pulse Rate

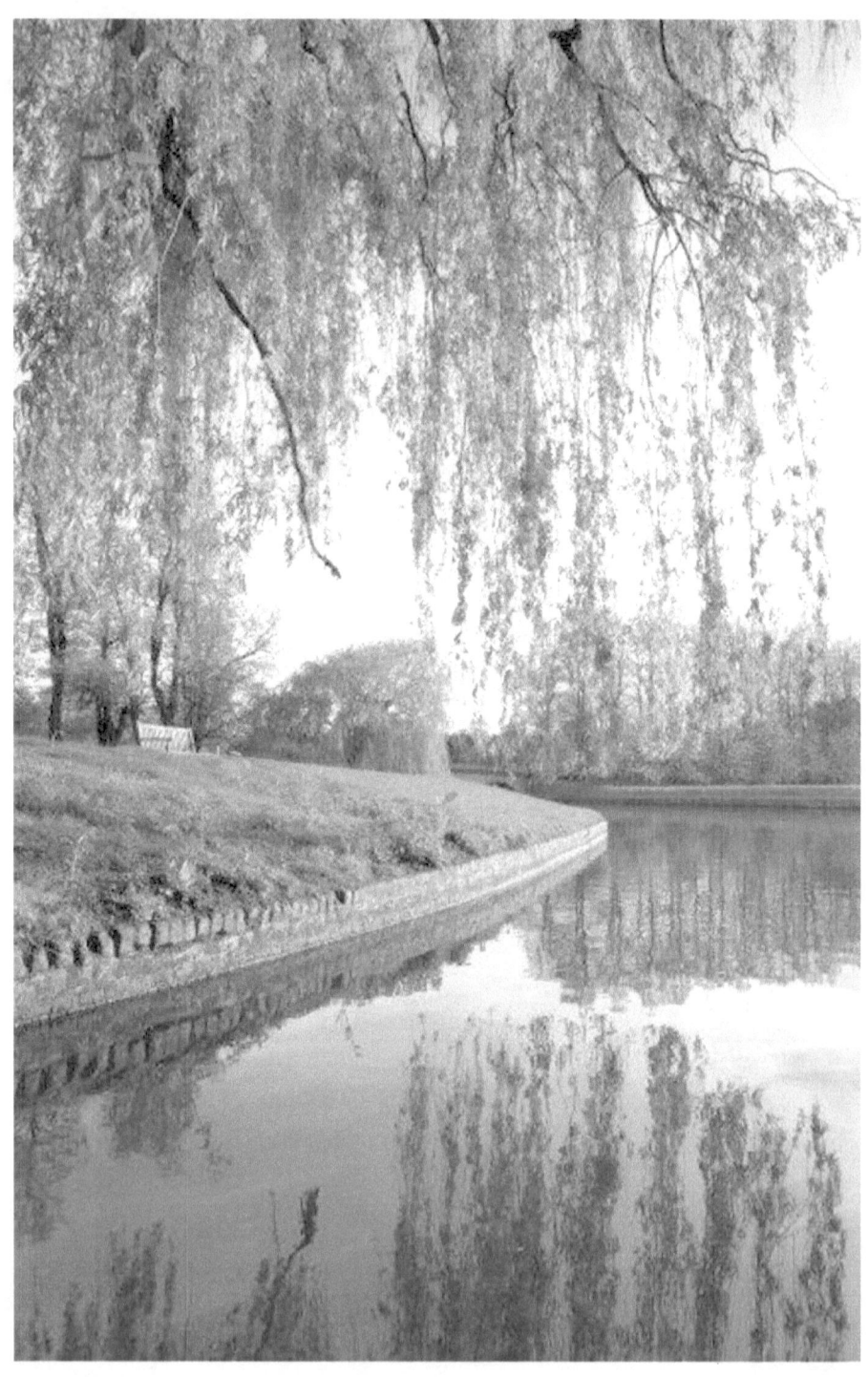

HYPERTENSION DIARY AND LOG

BLOOD PRESSURE LOG

Date / Day	Time	AM	PM	SYSTOLIC	DIASTOLIC	Pulse Rate

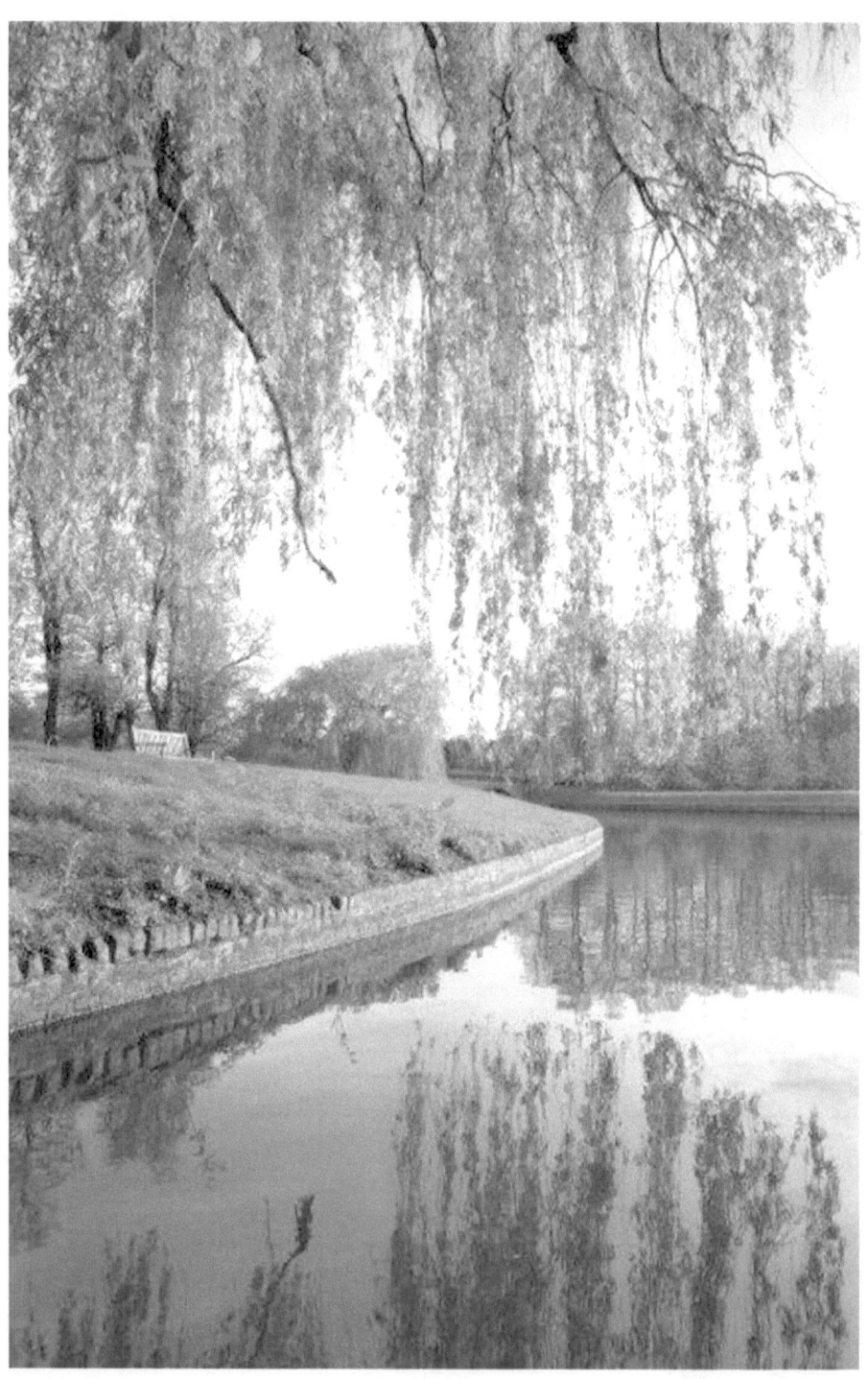

HYPERTENSION DIARY AND LOG

BLOOD PRESSURE LOG

Date / Day	Time	AM	PM	SYSTOLIC	DIASTOLIC	Pulse Rate

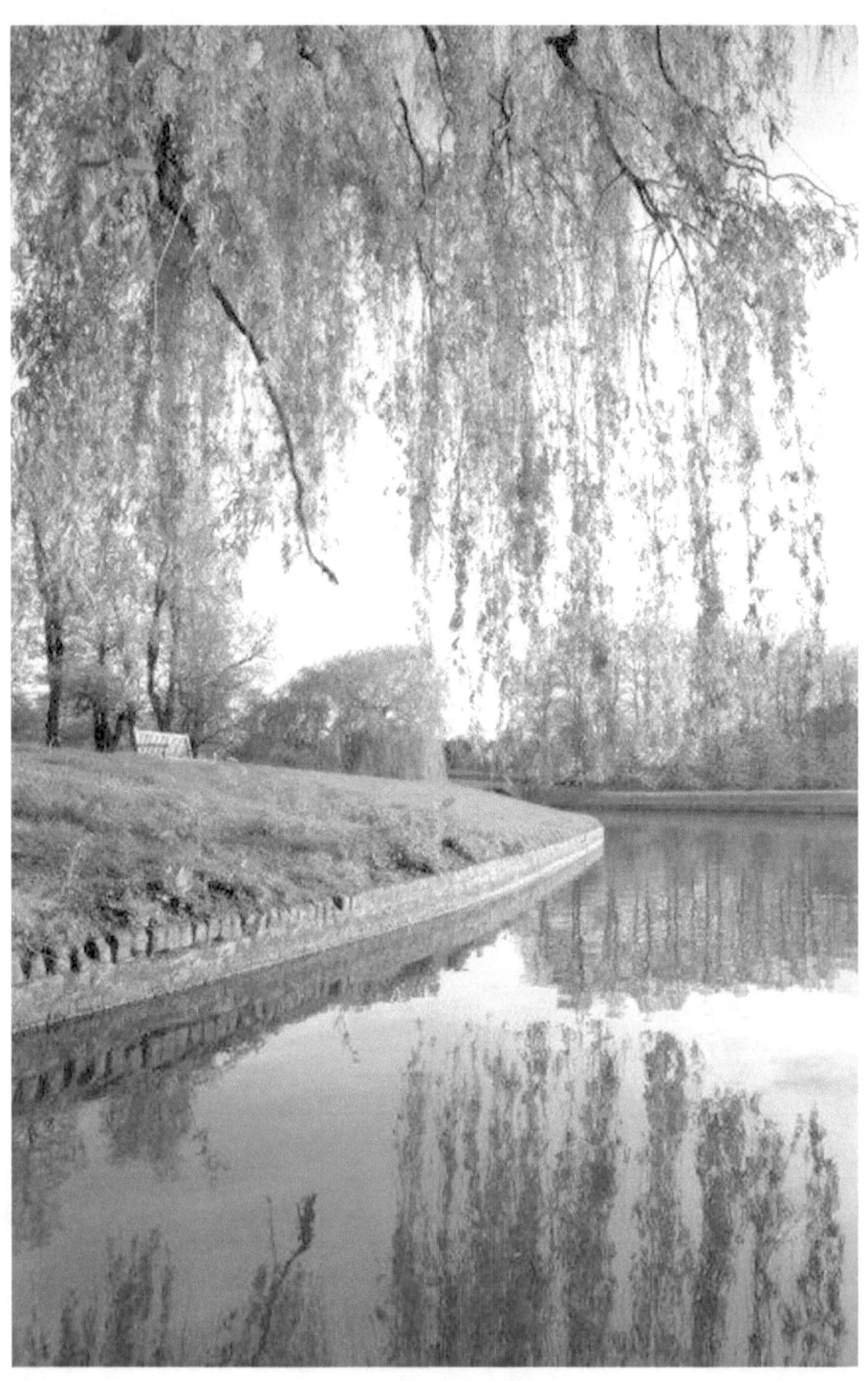

HYPERTENSION DIARY AND LOG

BLOOD PRESSURE LOG

Date / Day	Time	AM	PM	SYSTOLIC	DIASTOLIC	Pulse Rate

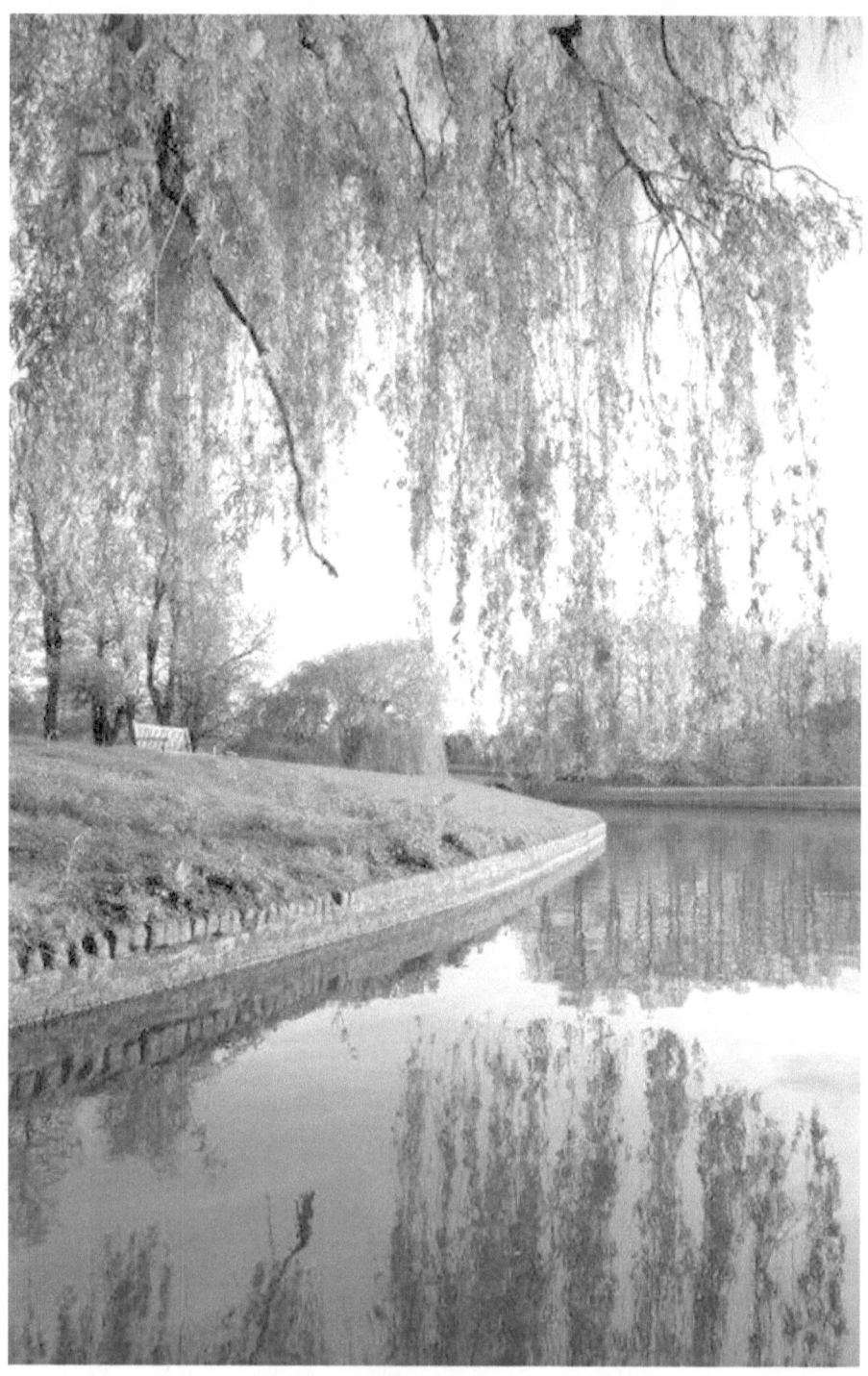

HYPERTENSION DIARY AND LOG

BLOOD PRESSURE LOG

Date / Day	Time	AM	PM	SYSTOLIC	DIASTOLIC	Pulse Rate

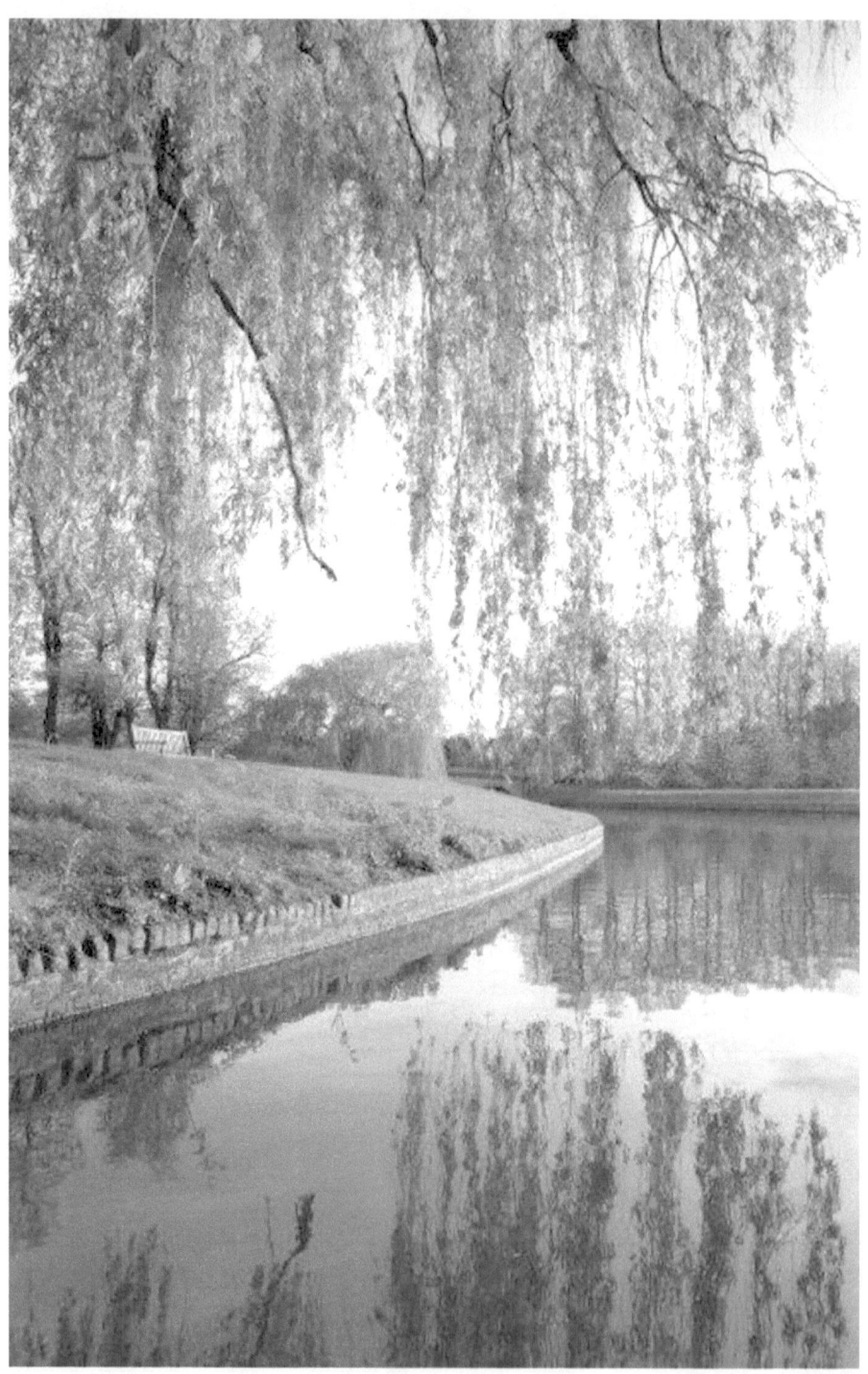

HYPERTENSION DIARY AND LOG

BLOOD PRESSURE LOG

Date / Day	Time	AM	PM	SYSTOLIC	DIASTOLIC	Pulse Rate

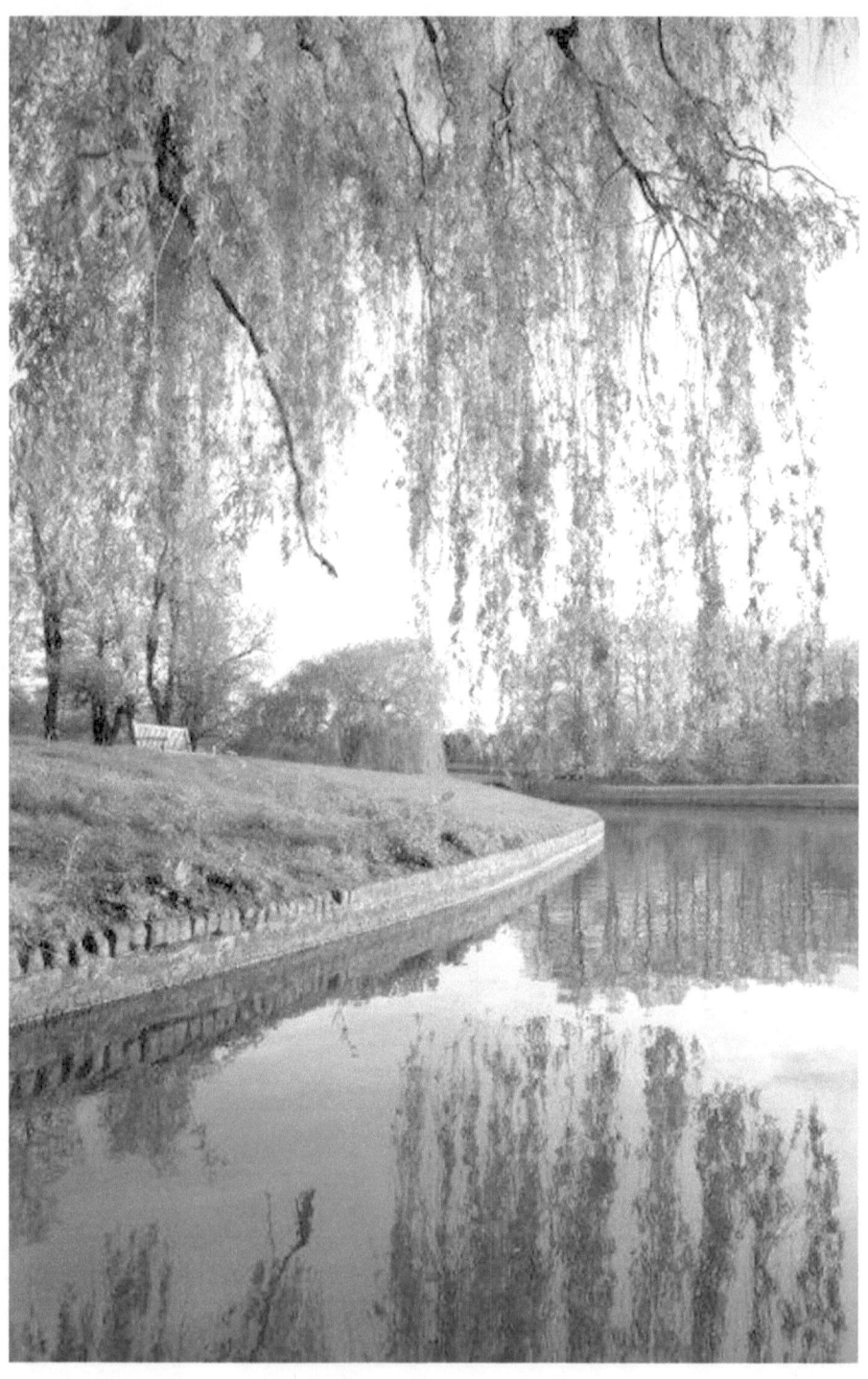

BLOOD PRESSURE LOG

Date / Day	Time	AM	PM	SYSTOLIC	DIASTOLIC	Pulse Rate

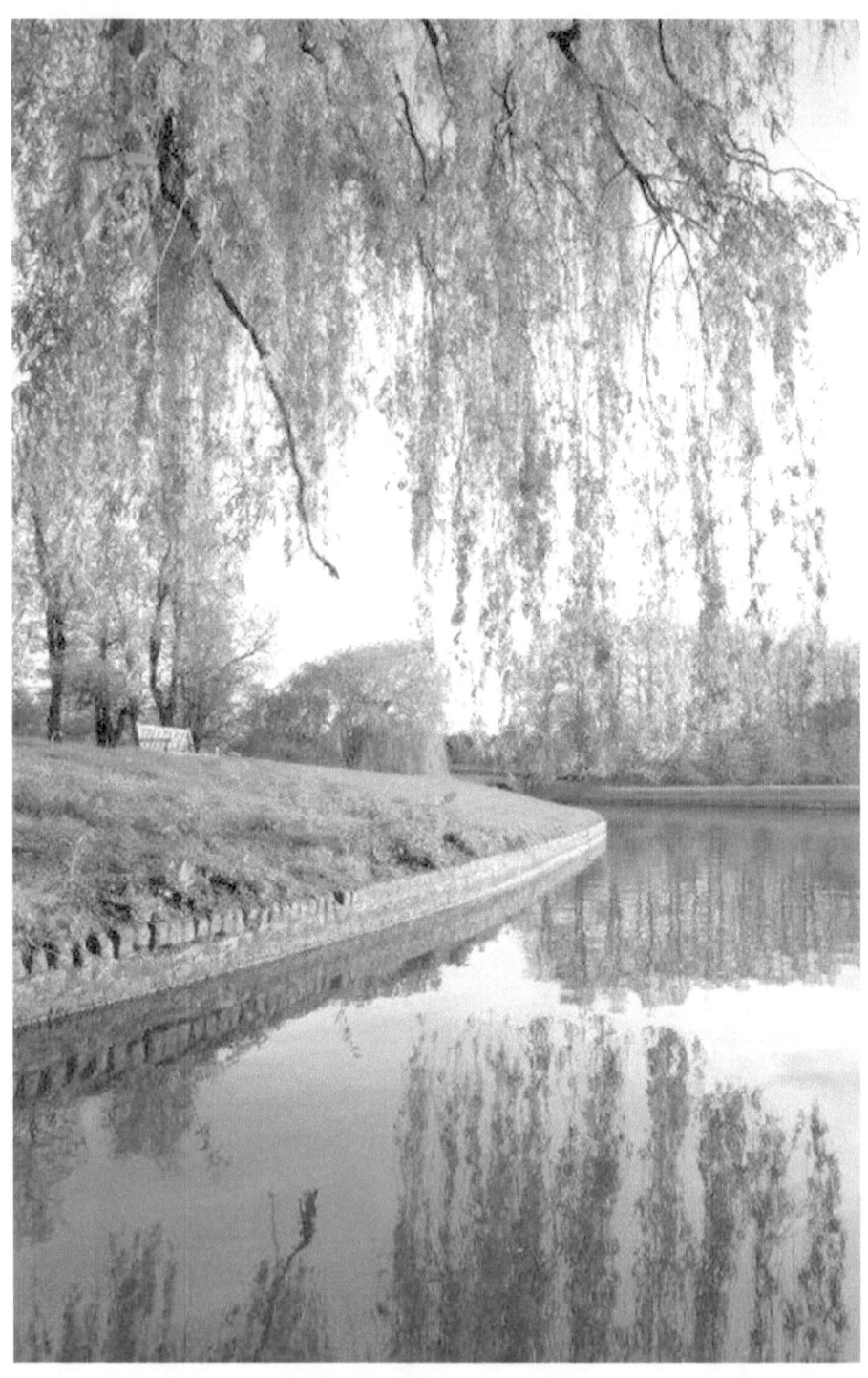

HYPERTENSION DIARY AND LOG

NUTRITION LOG

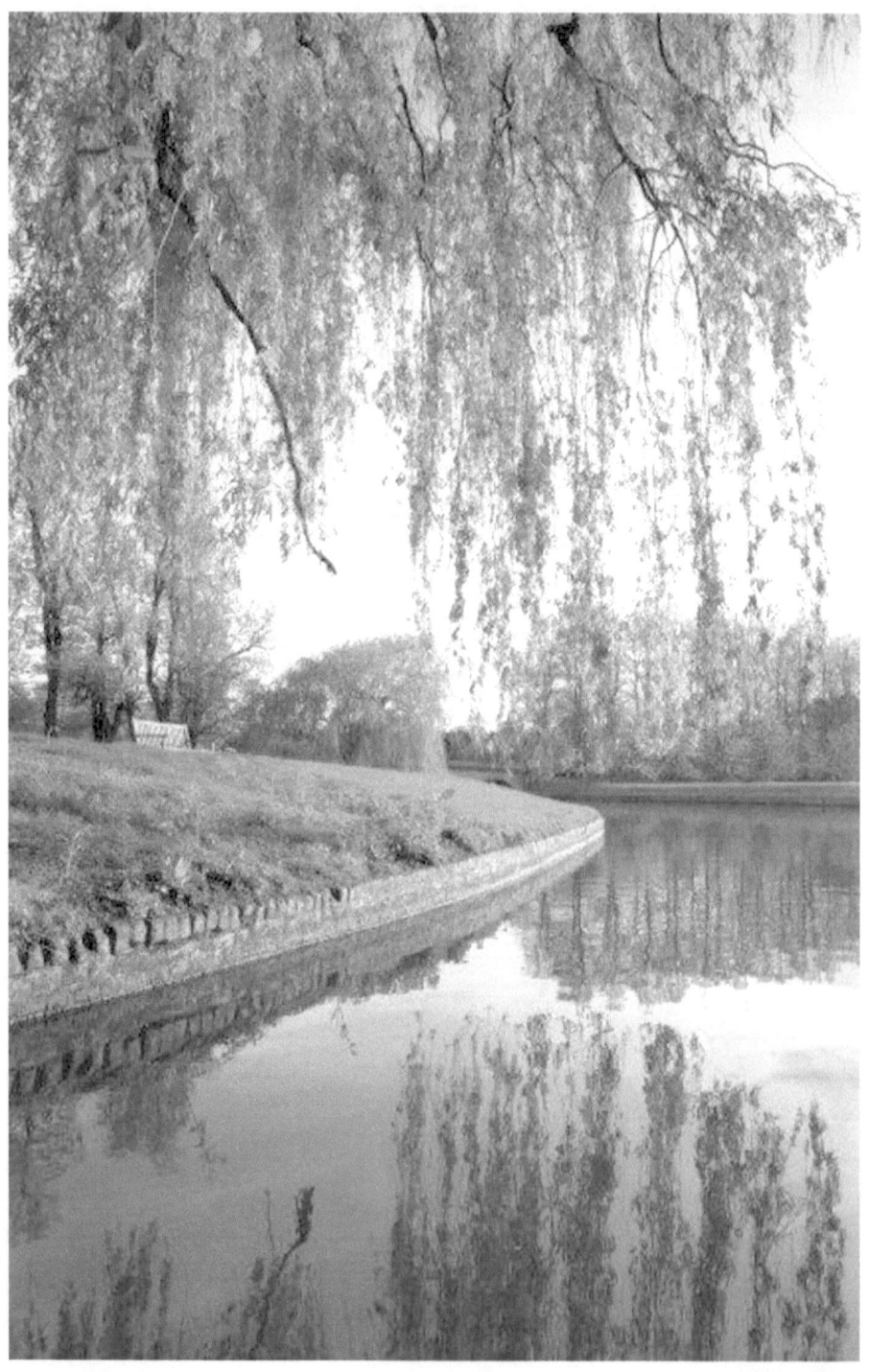

HYPERTENSION DIARY AND LOG

NUTRITION LOG

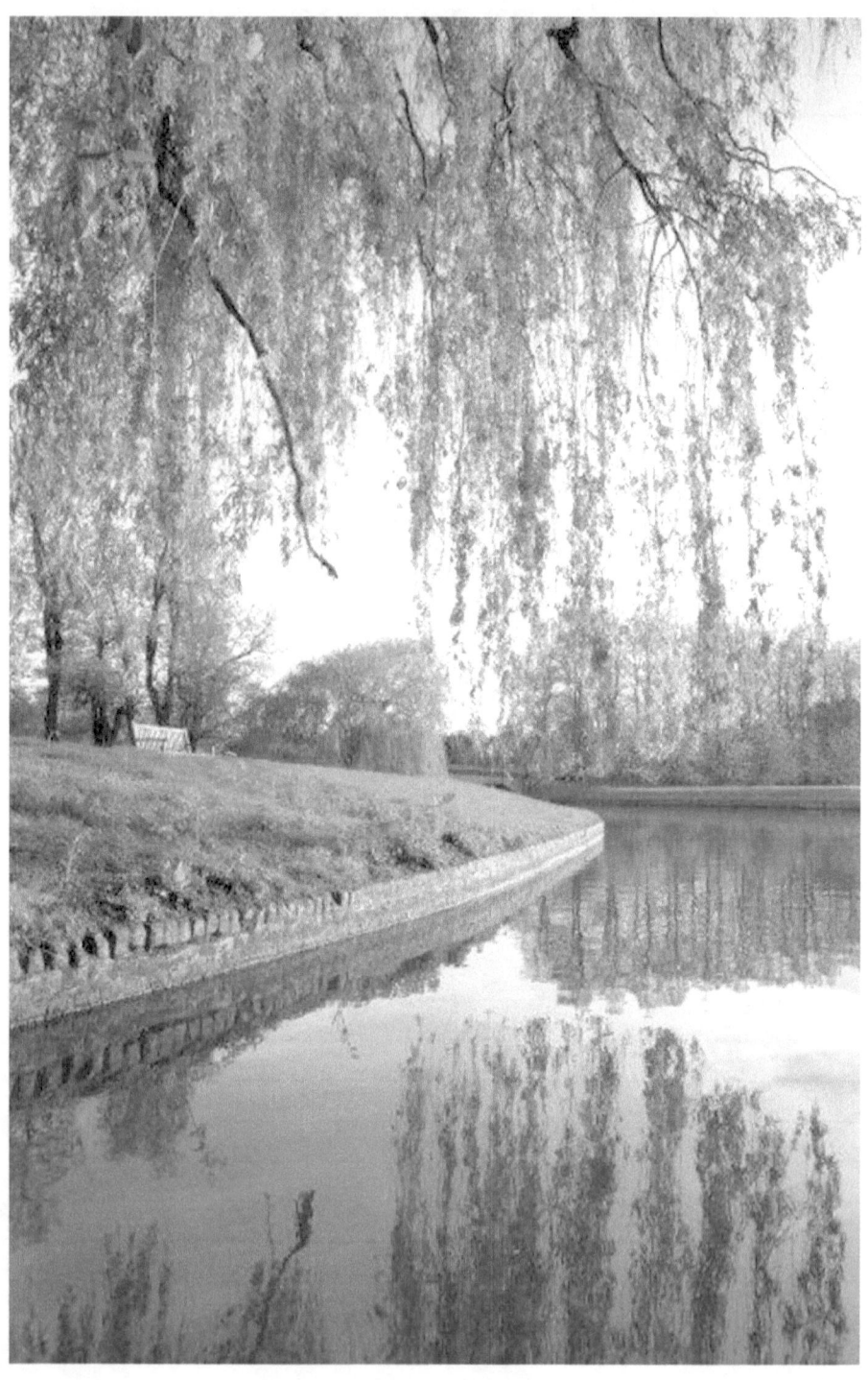

HYPERTENSION DIARY AND LOG

NUTRITION LOG

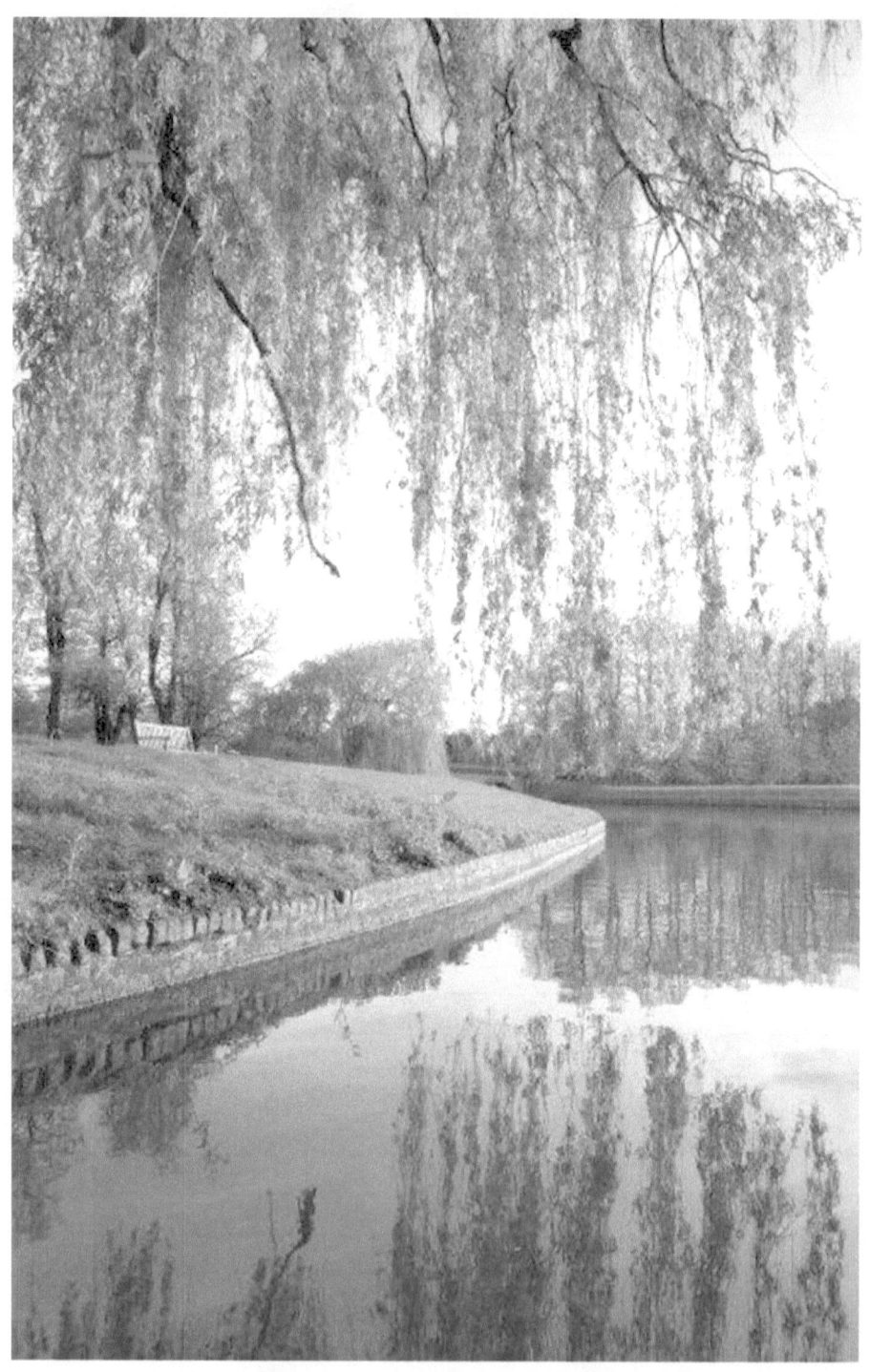

HYPERTENSION DIARY AND LOG

NUTRITION LOG

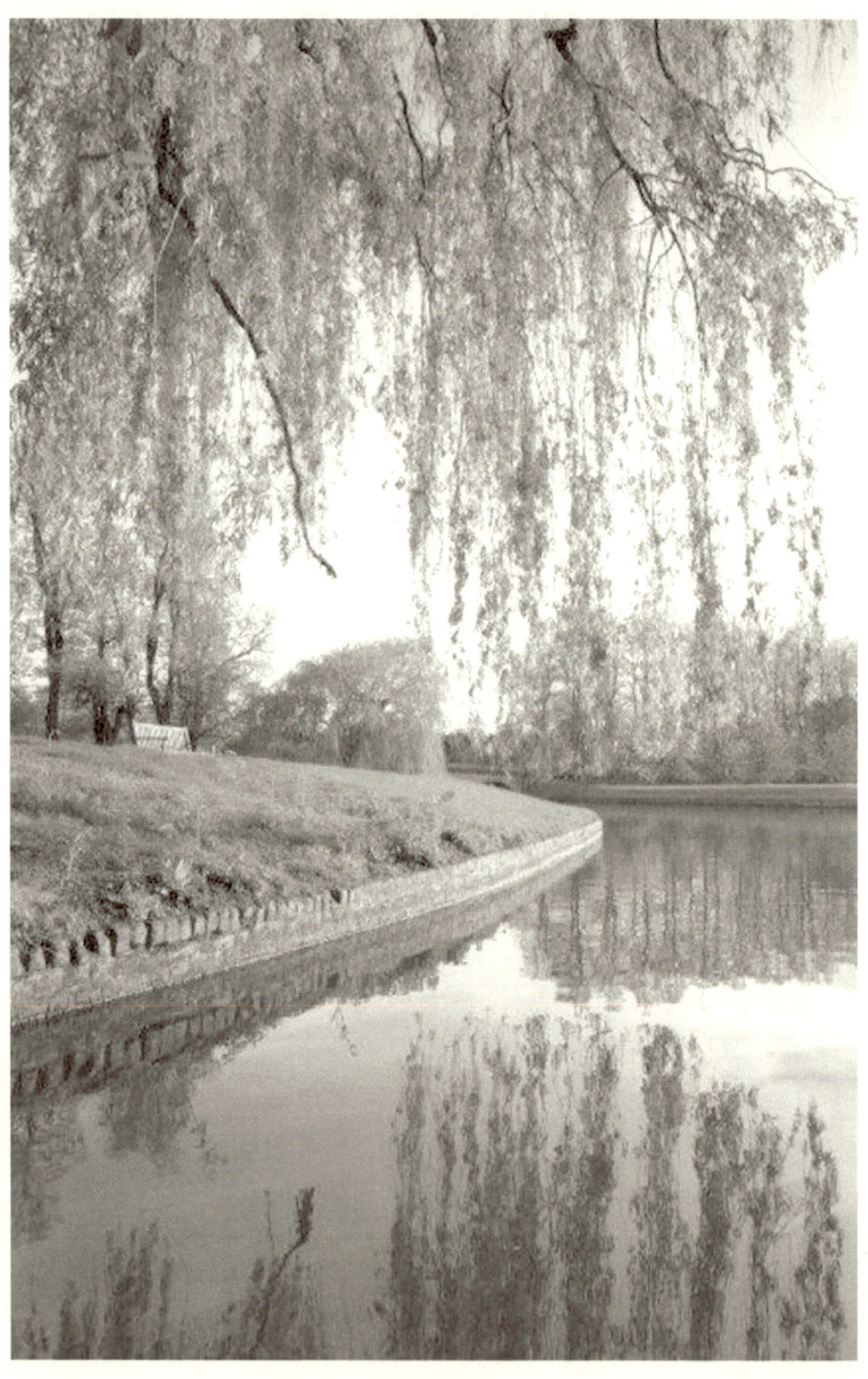

NUTRITION LOG

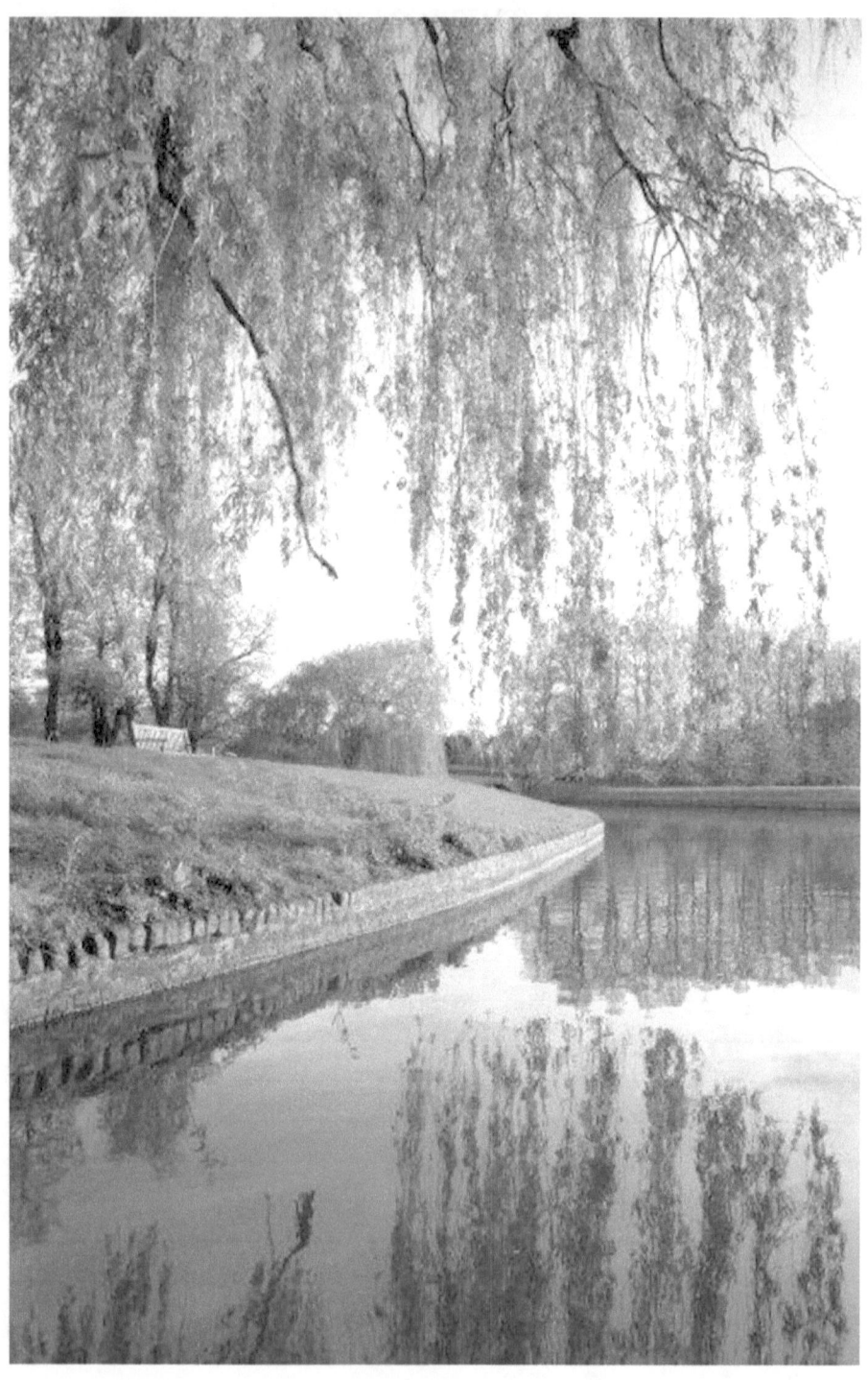

HYPERTENSION DIARY AND LOG

NUTRITION LOG

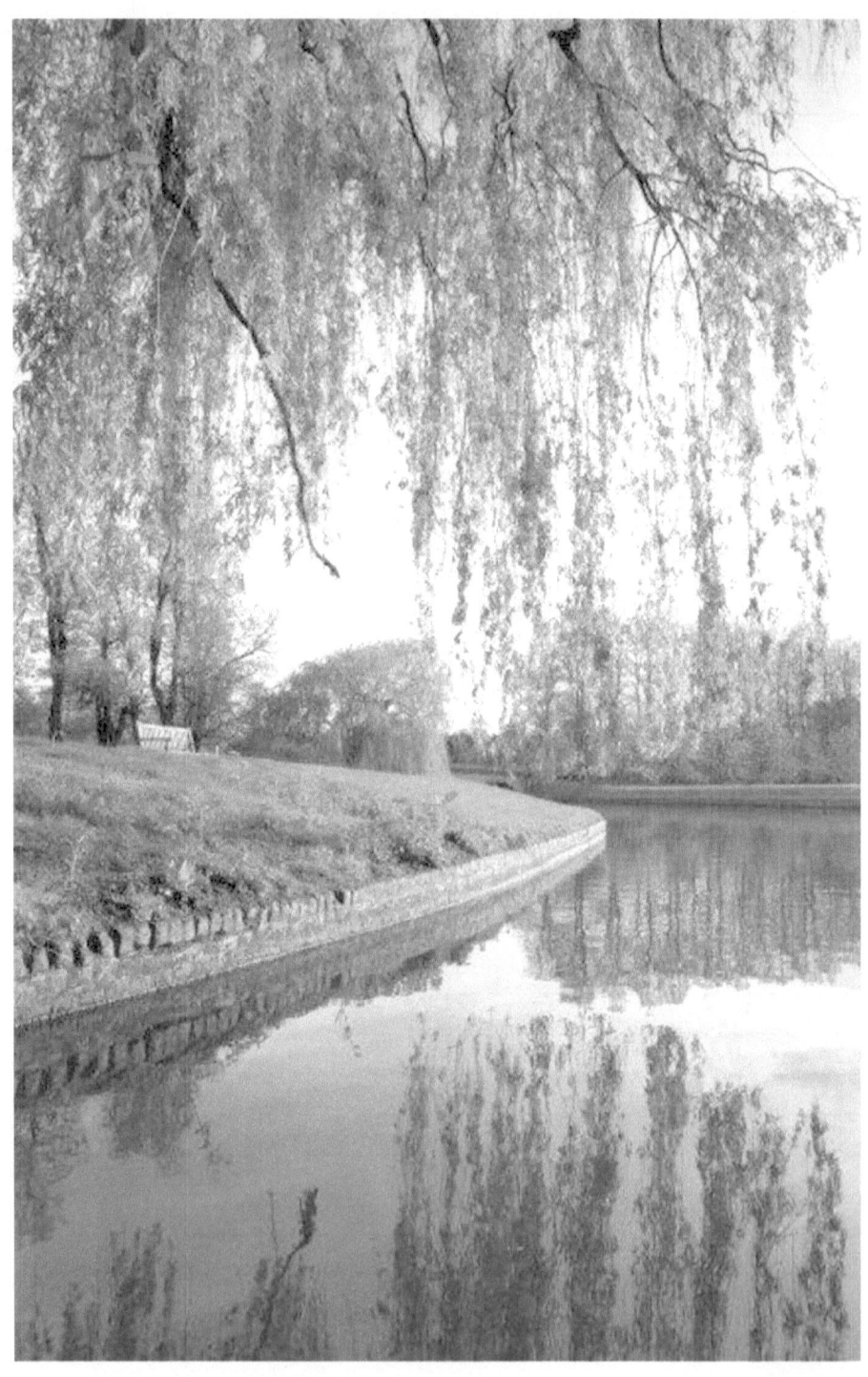

HYPERTENSION DIARY AND LOG

NUTRITION LOG

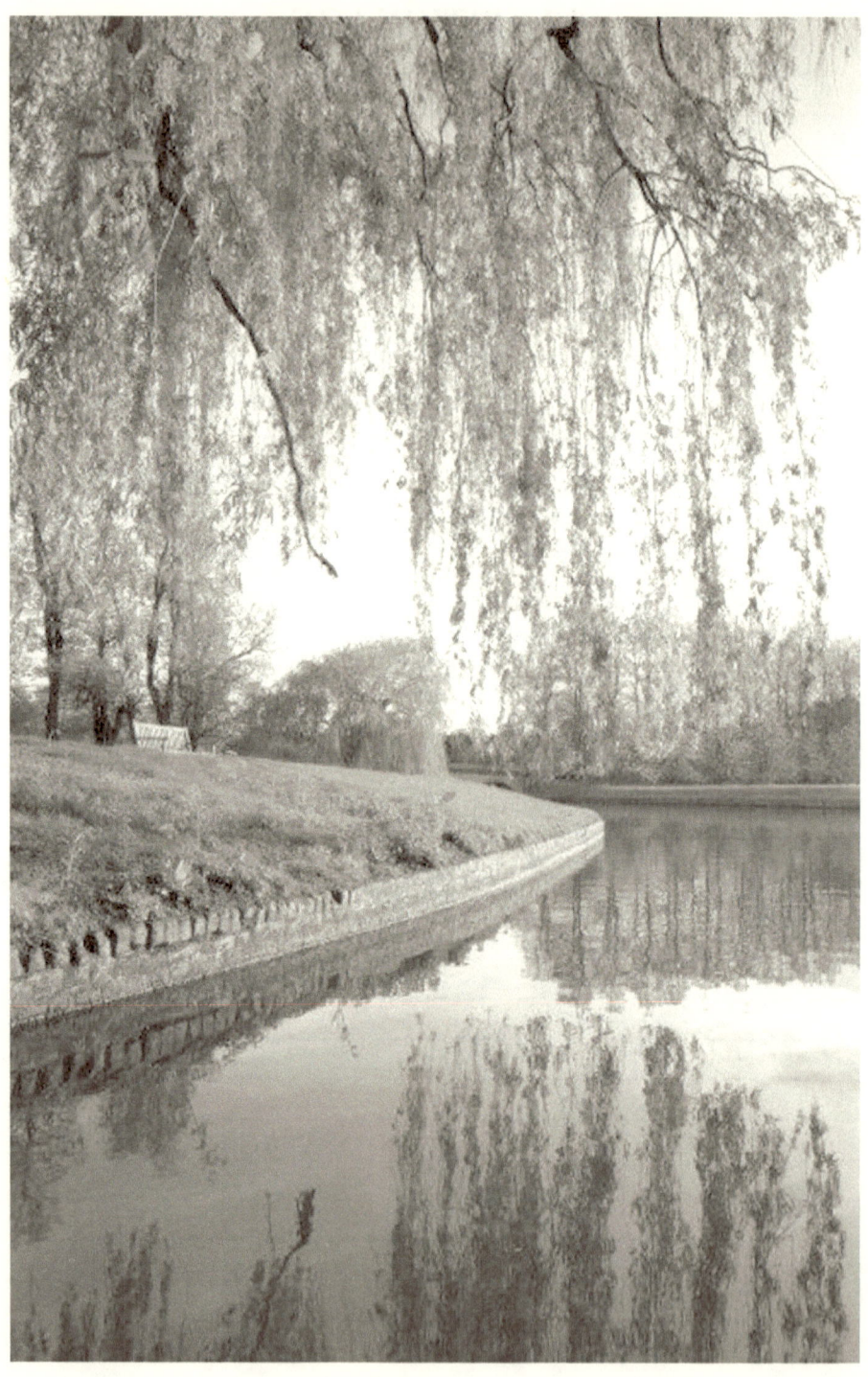

NUTRITION LOG

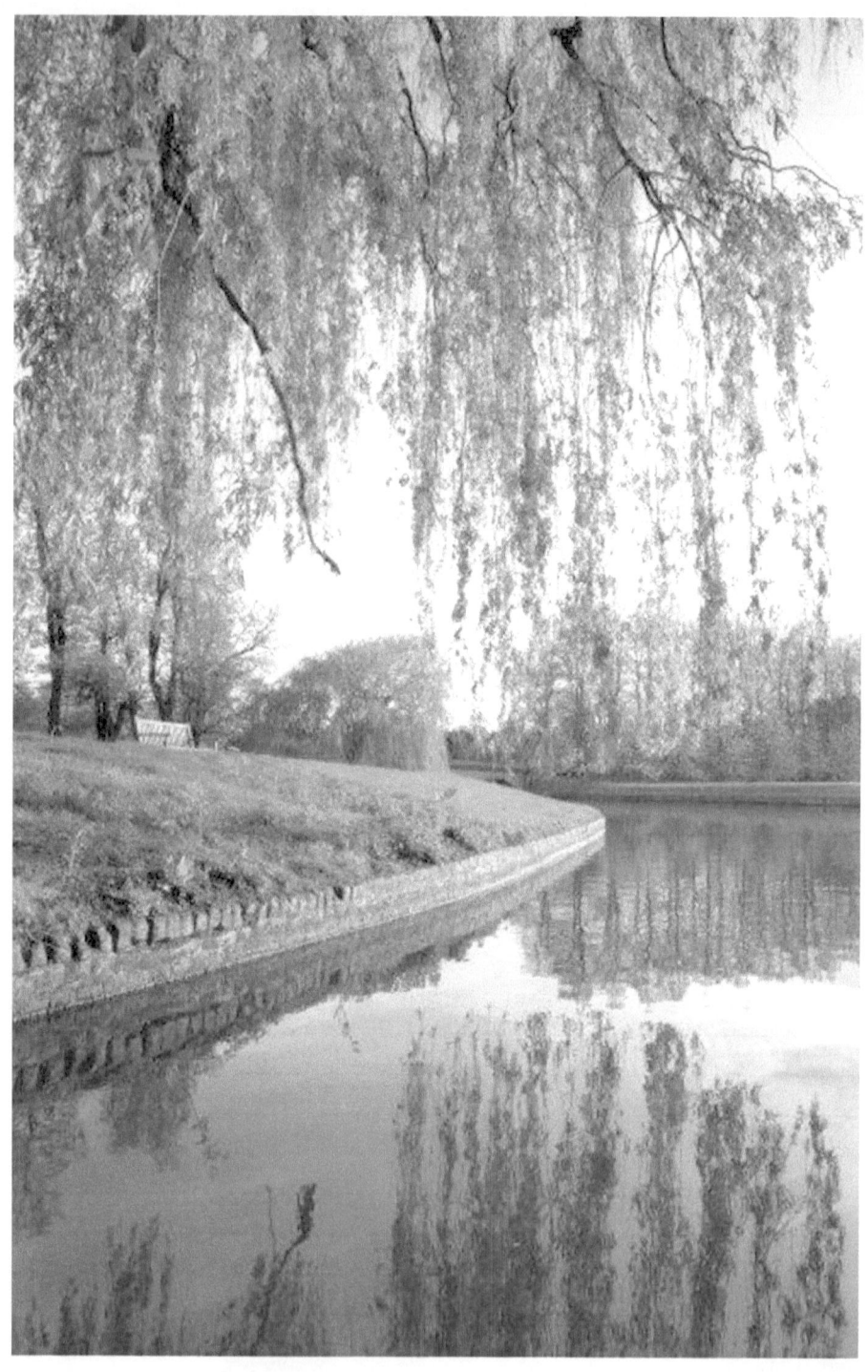

HYPERTENSION DIARY AND LOG

NUTRITION LOG

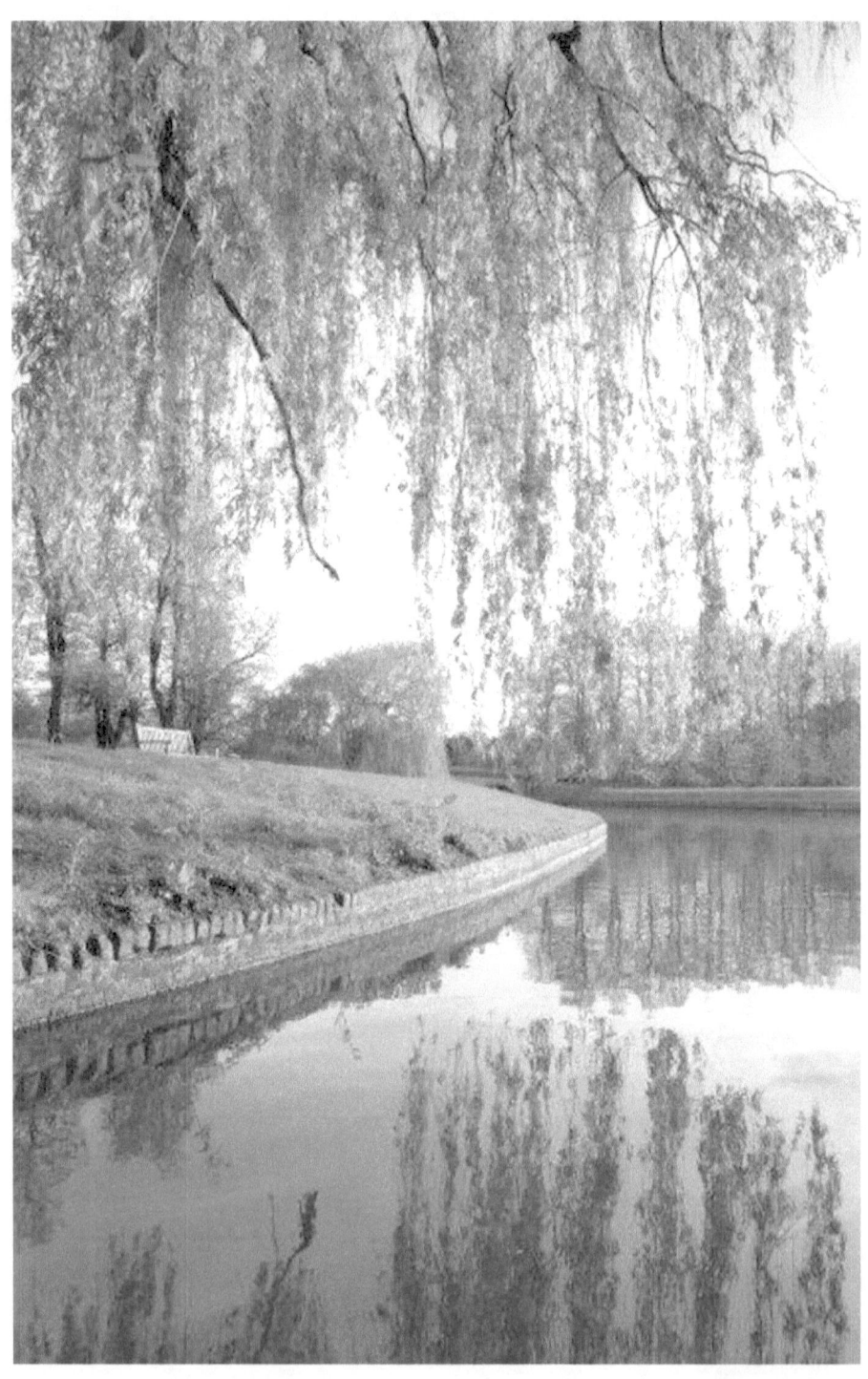

HYPERTENSION DIARY AND LOG

NUTRITION LOG

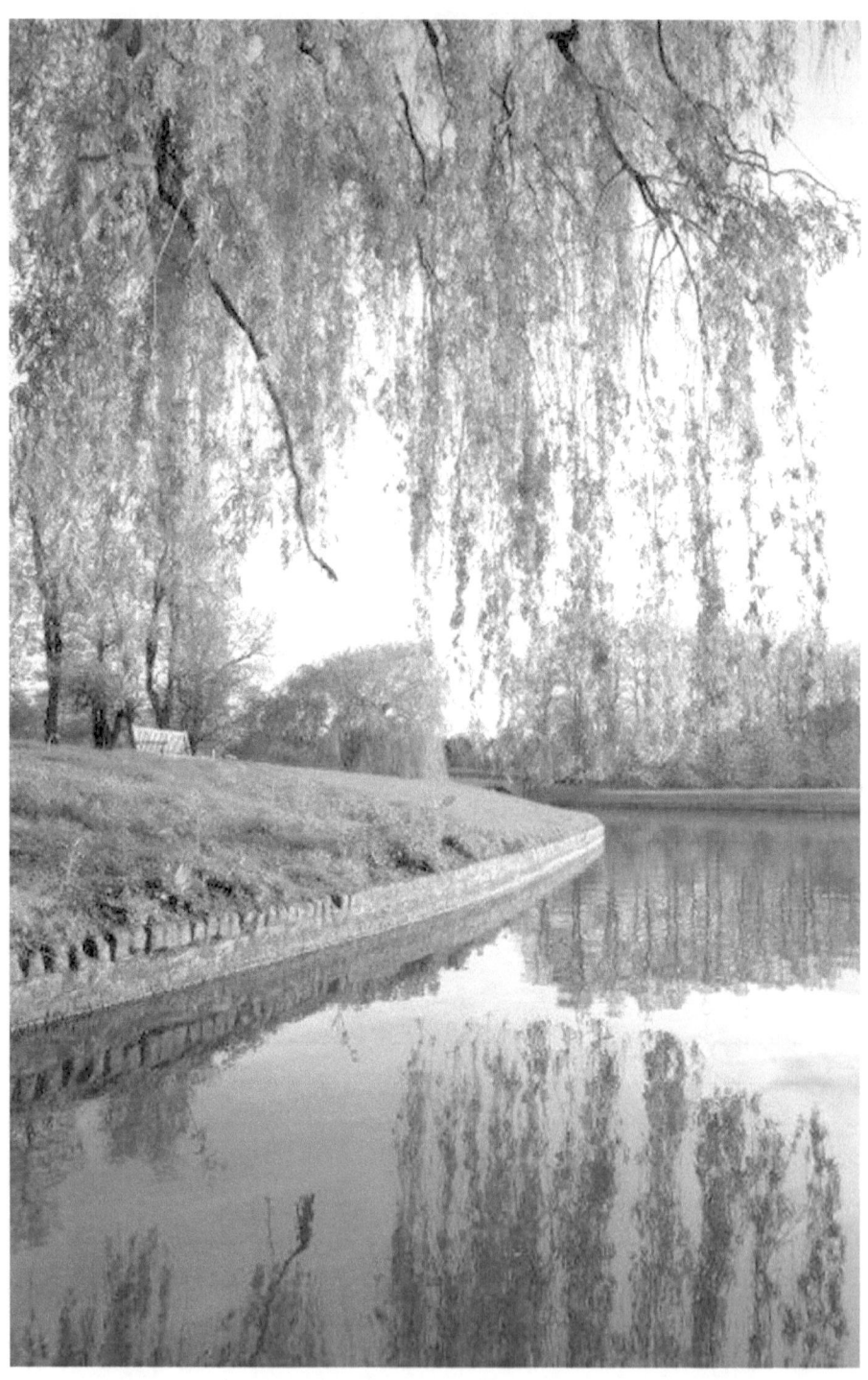

HYPERTENSION DIARY AND LOG

NUTRITION LOG

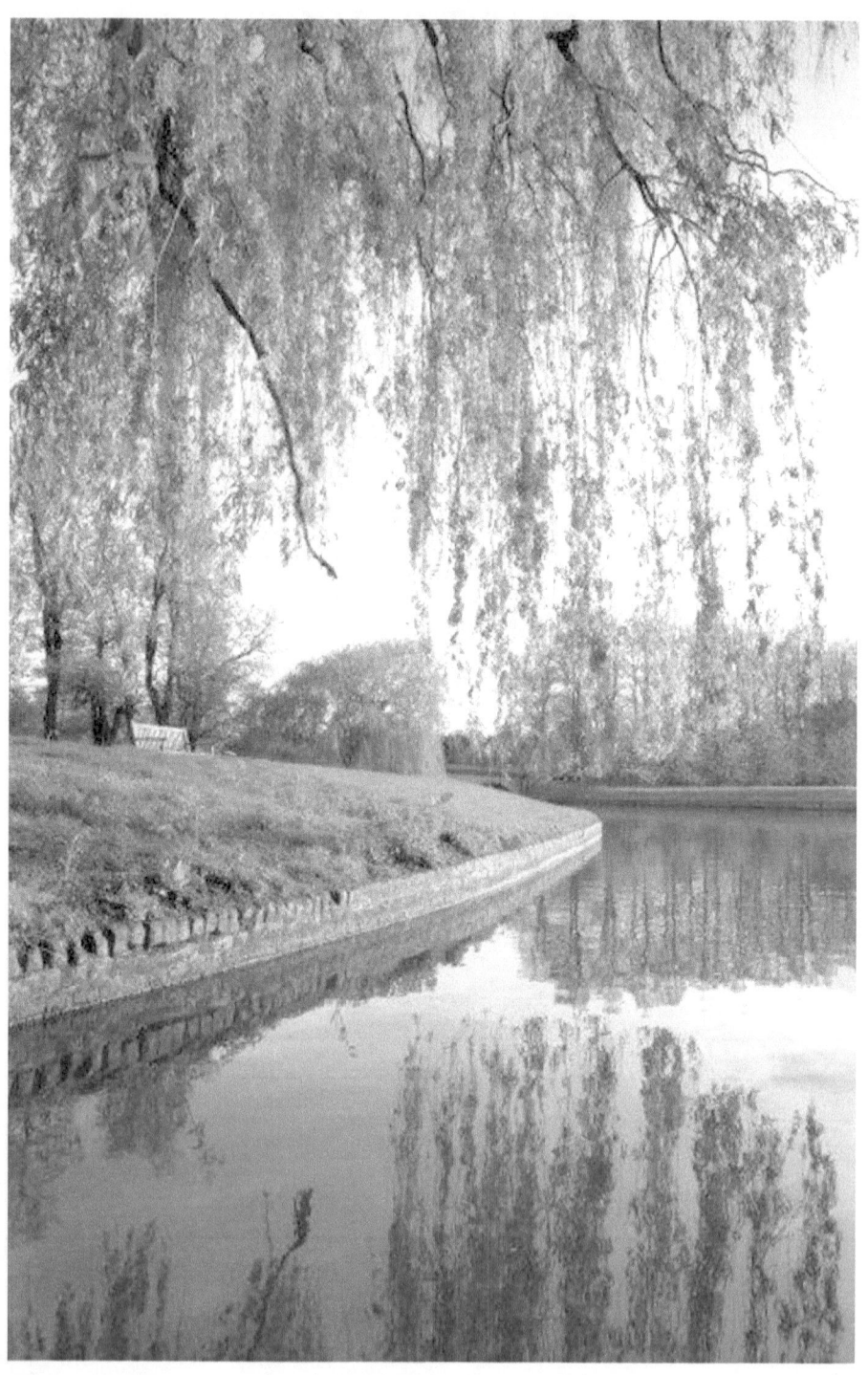

NUTRITION LOG

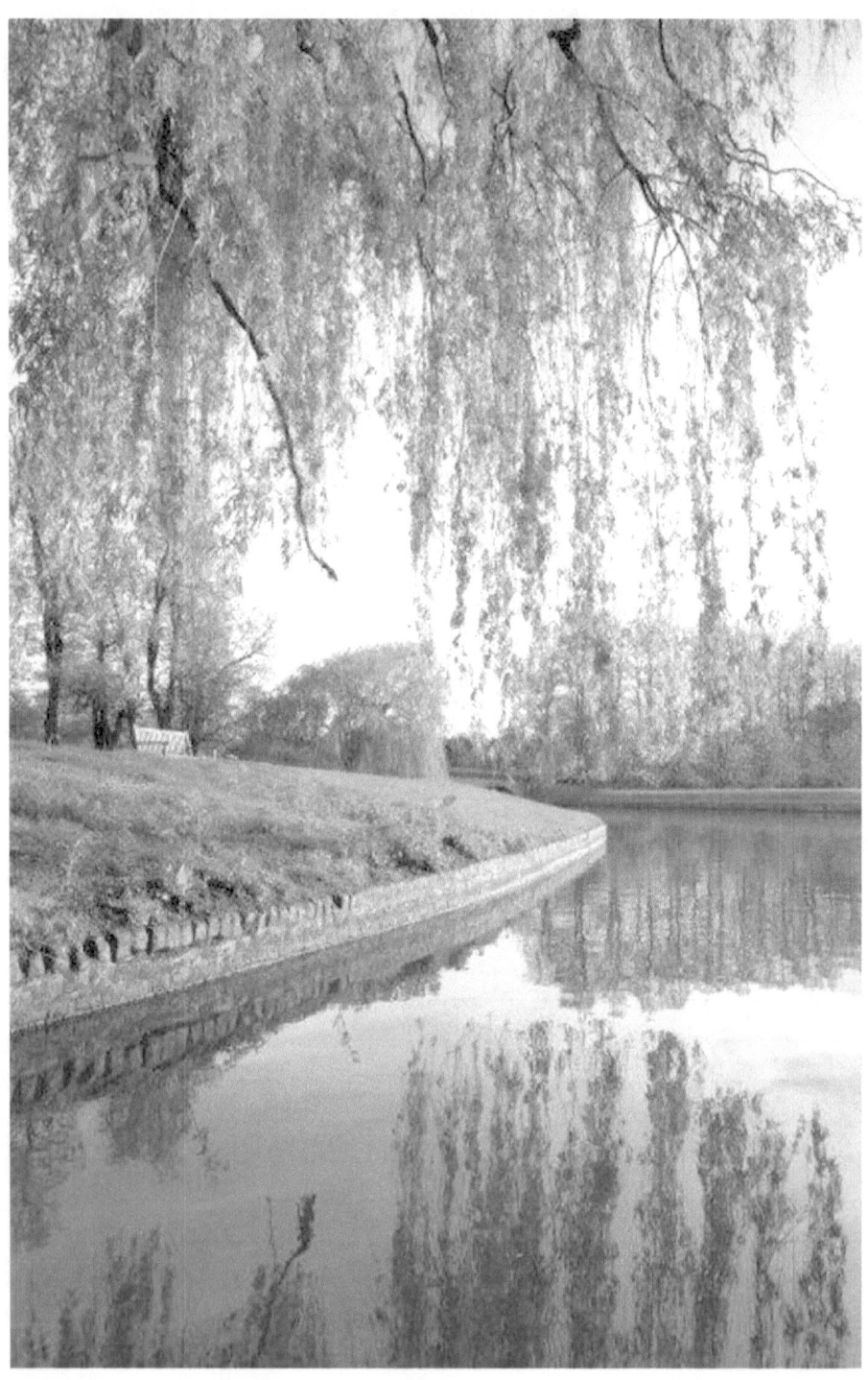

HYPERTENSION DIARY AND LOG

NUTRITION LOG

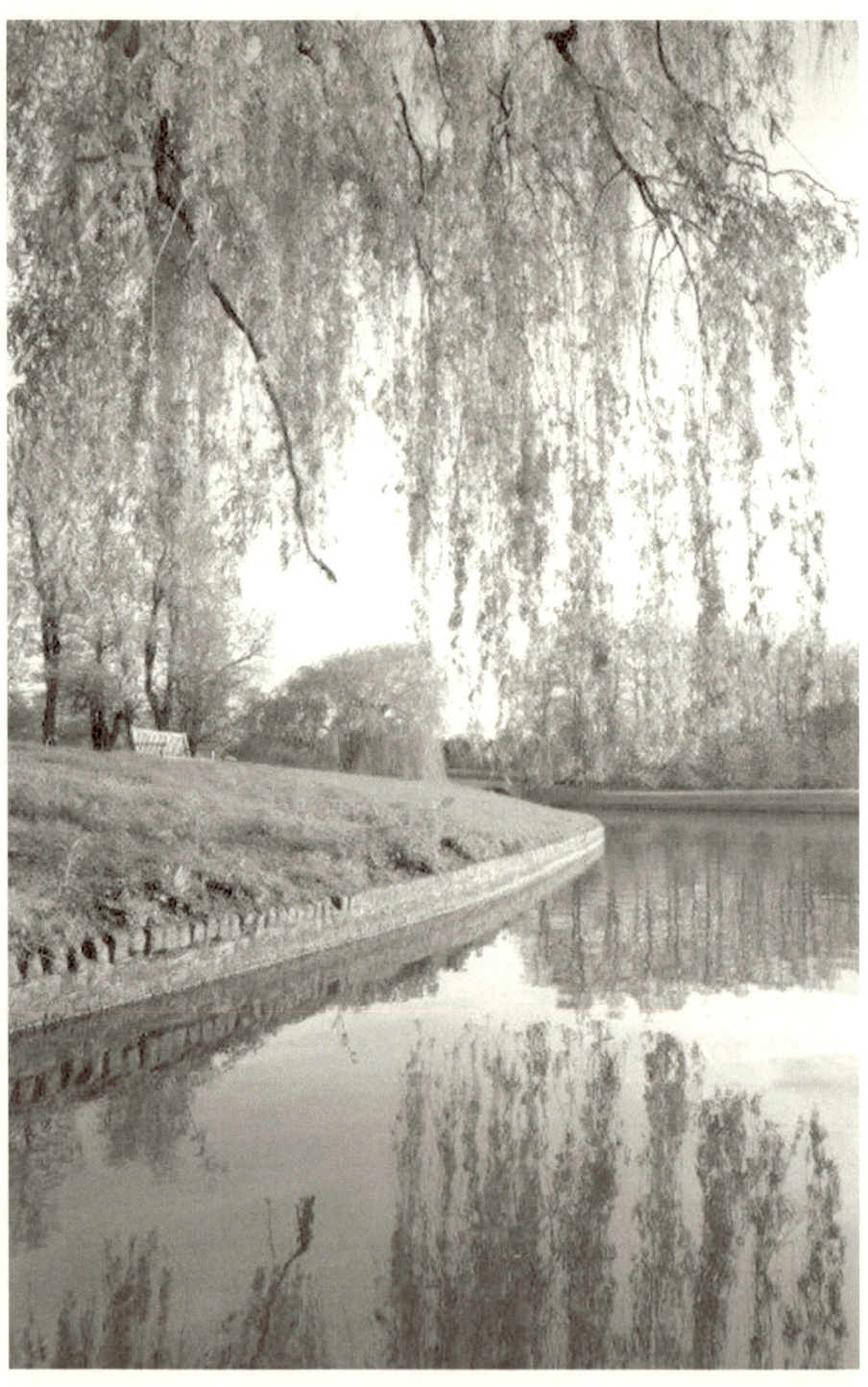

HYPERTENSION DIARY AND LOG

NUTRITION LOG

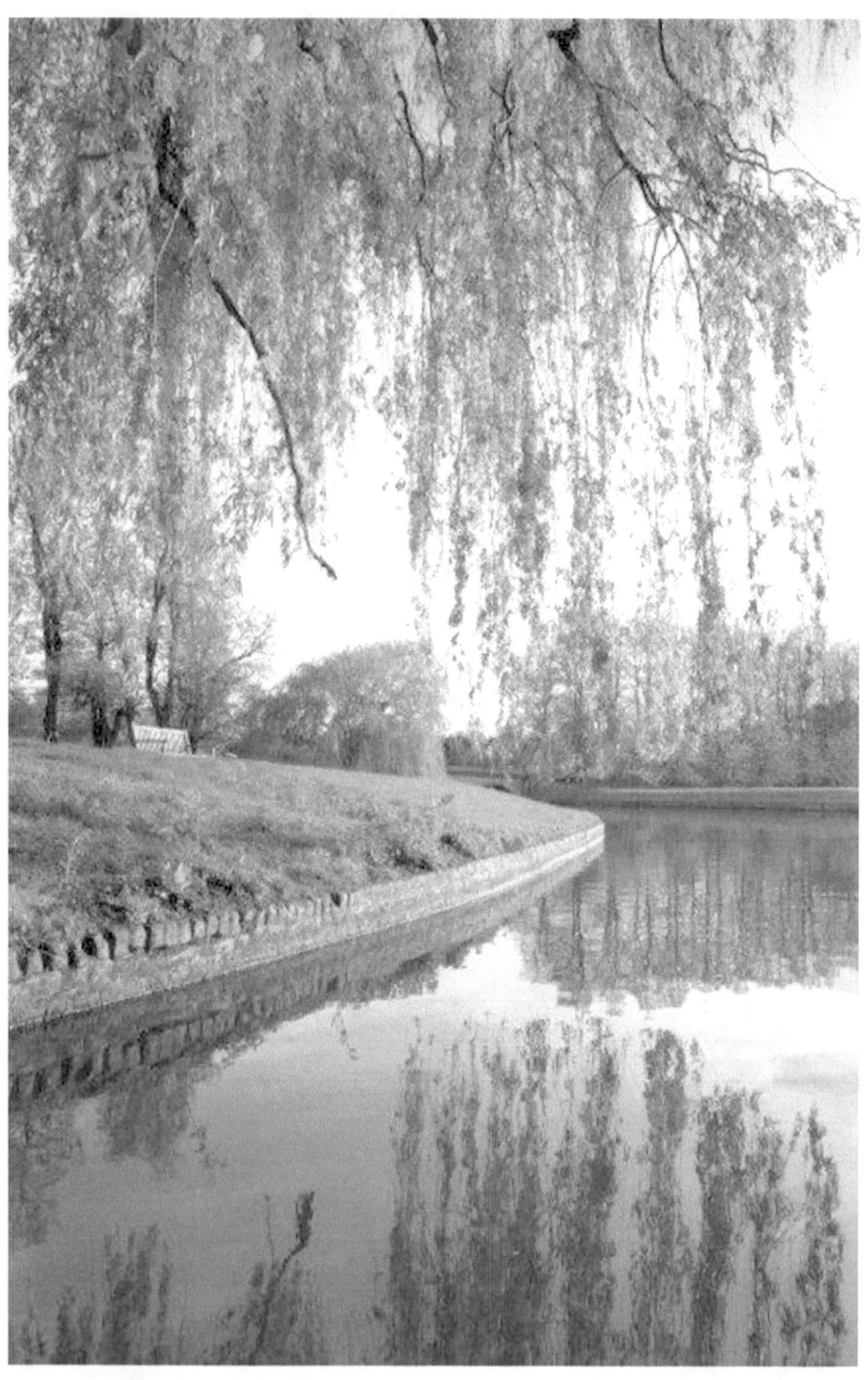

HYPERTENSION DIARY AND LOG

NUTRITION LOG

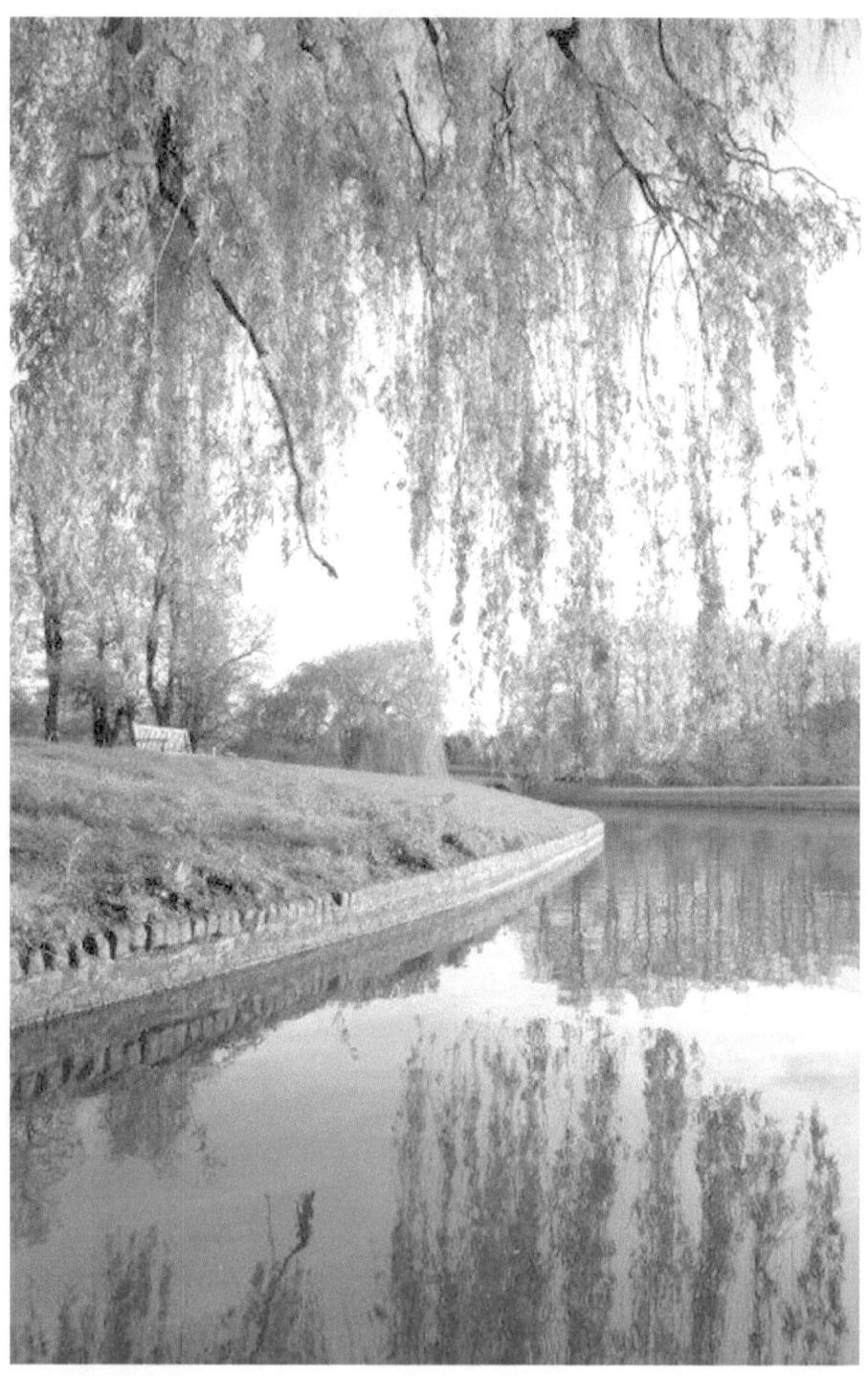

HYPERTENSION DIARY AND LOG

ACTIVITY LOG

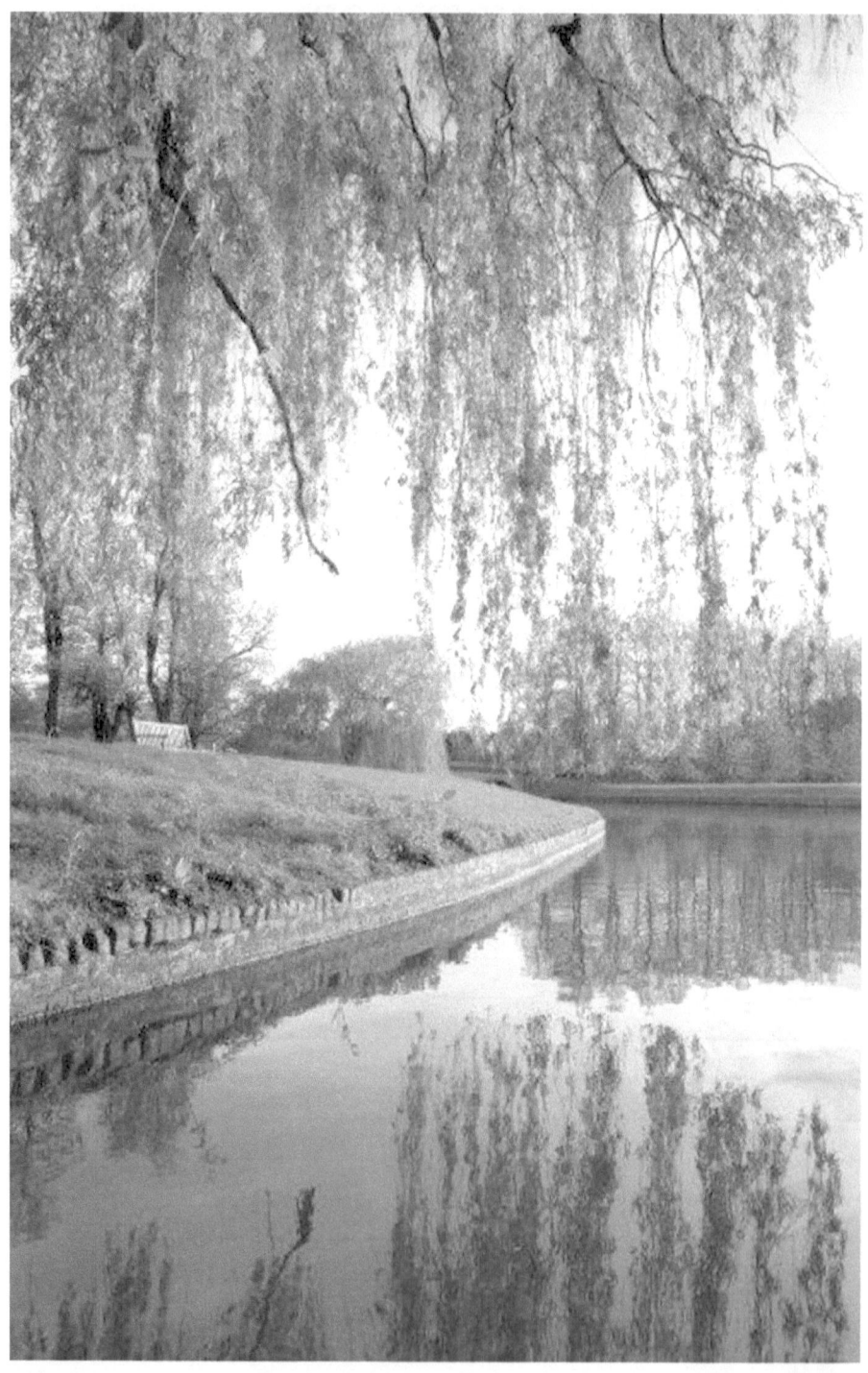

HYPERTENSION DIARY AND LOG

ACTIVITY LOG

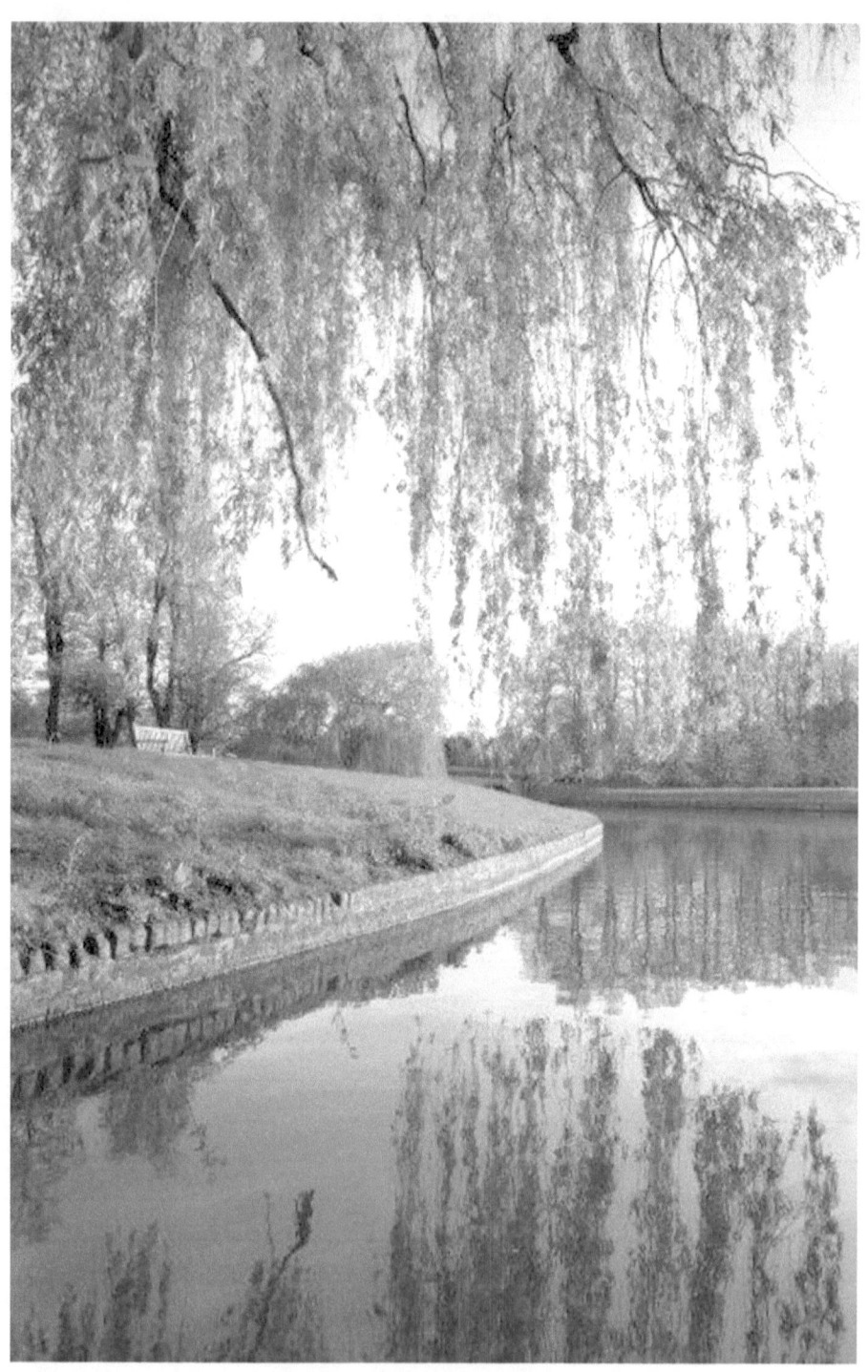

HYPERTENSION DIARY AND LOG

ACTIVITY LOG

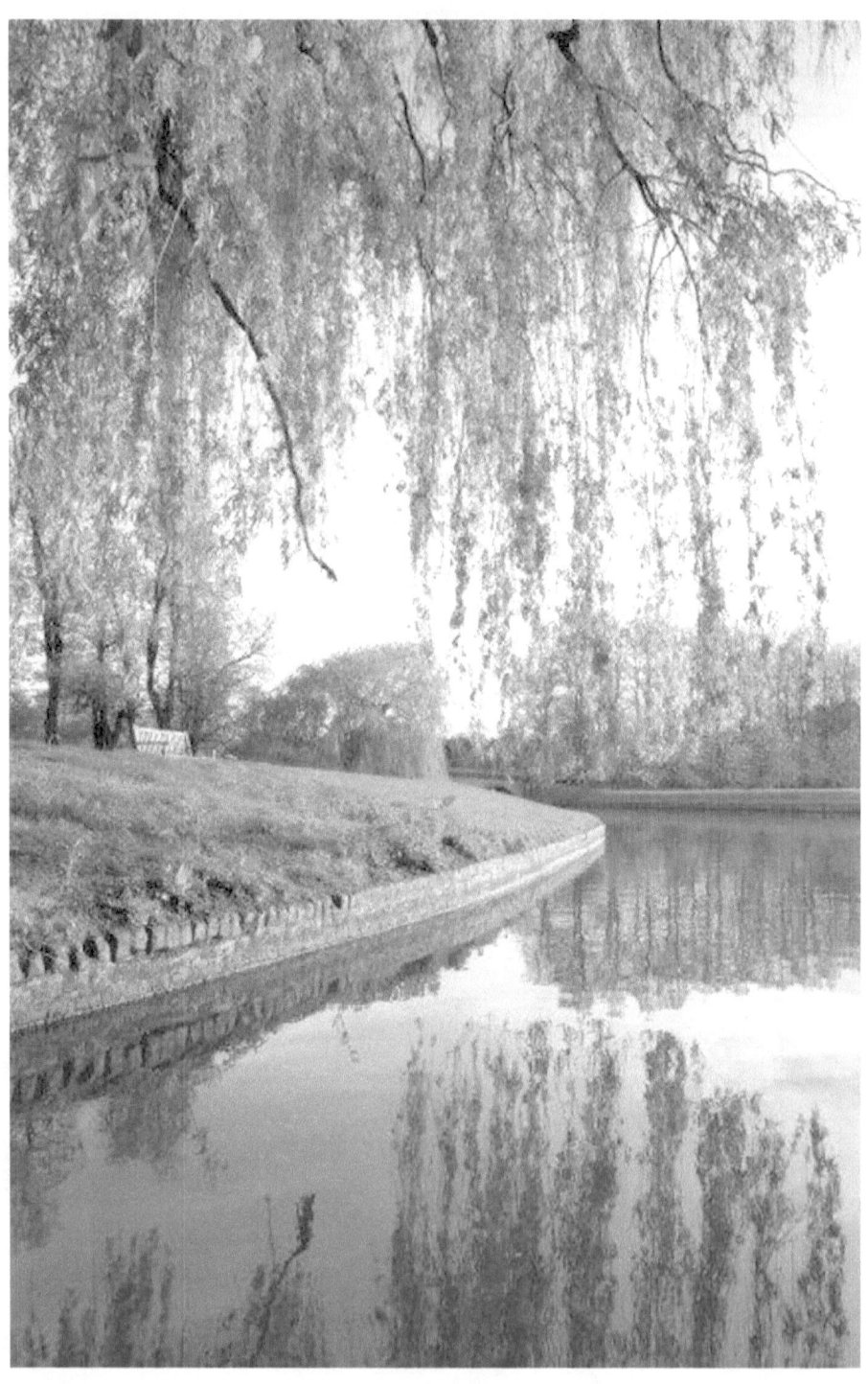

HYPERTENSION DIARY AND LOG

ACTIVITY LOG

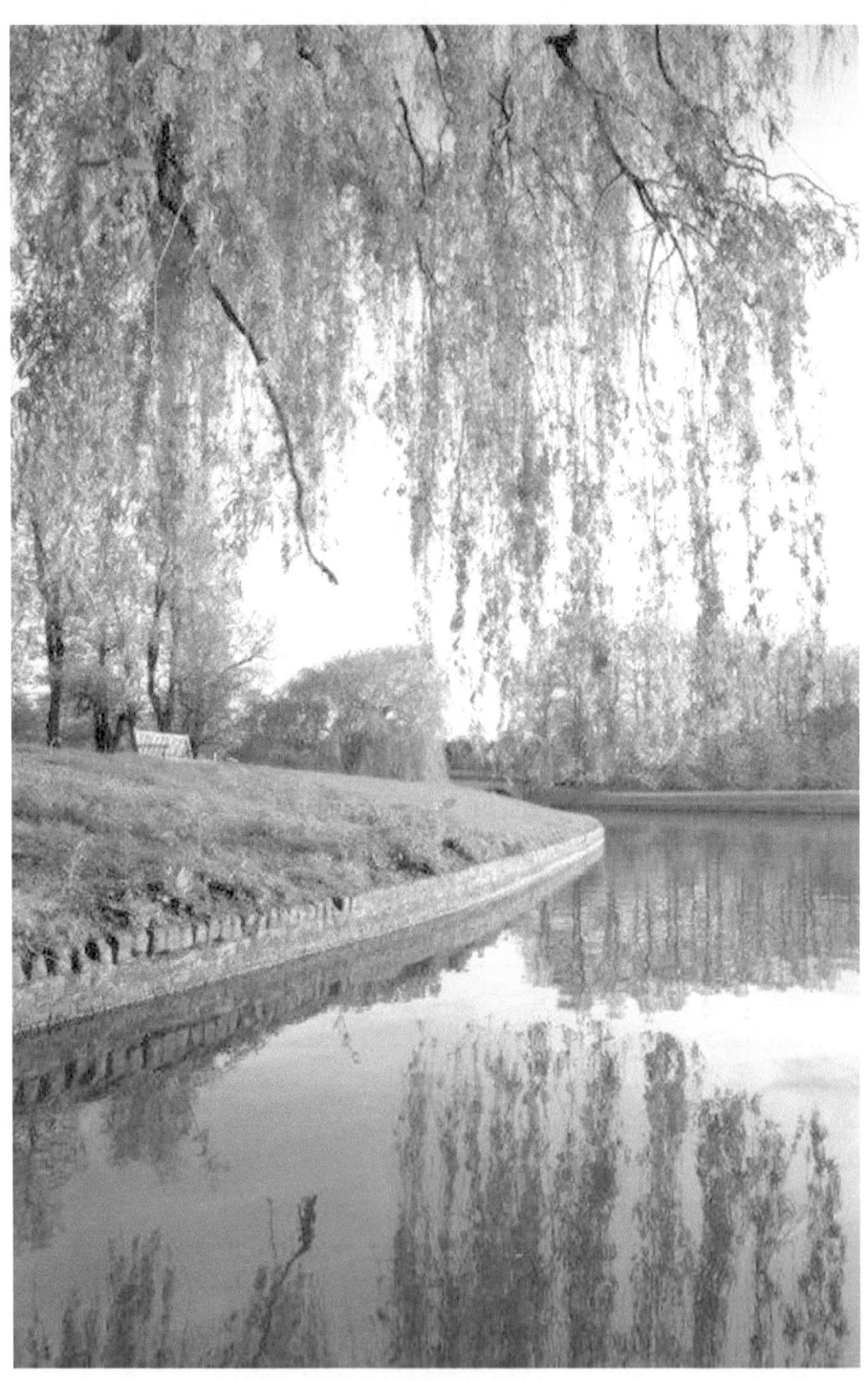

HYPERTENSION DIARY AND LOG

ACTIVITY LOG

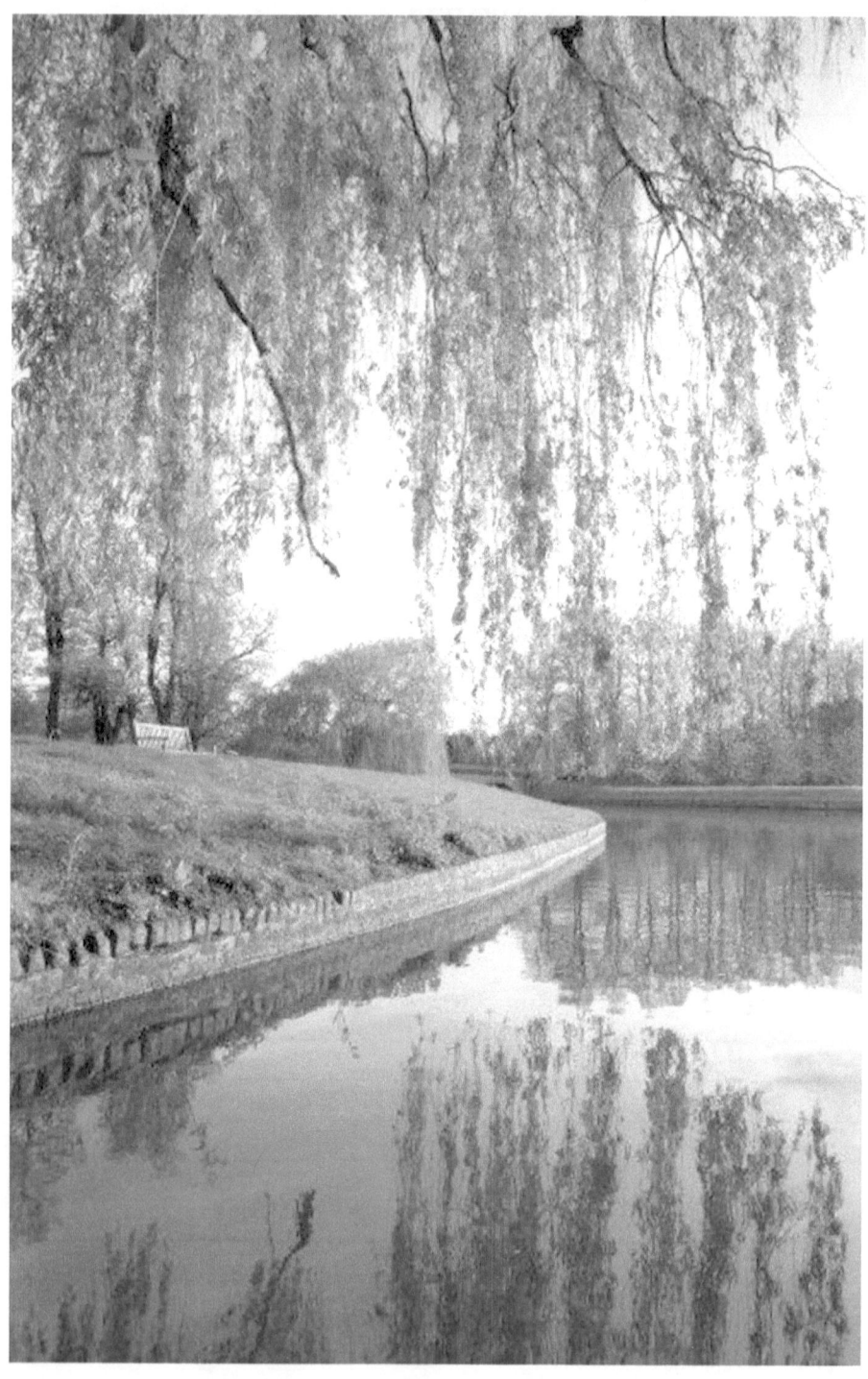

HYPERTENSION DIARY AND LOG

ACTIVITY LOG

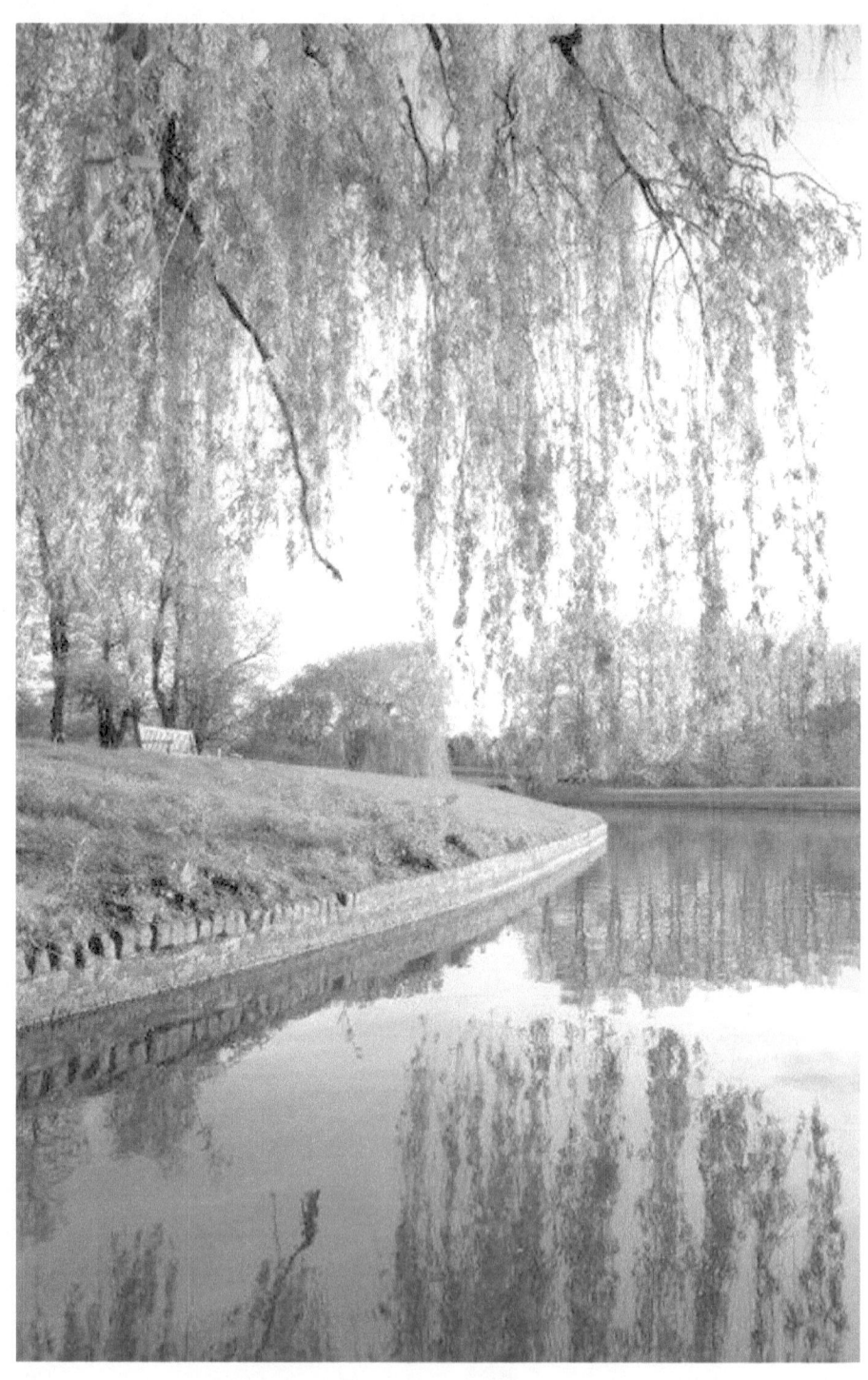

HYPERTENSION DIARY AND LOG

ACTIVITY LOG

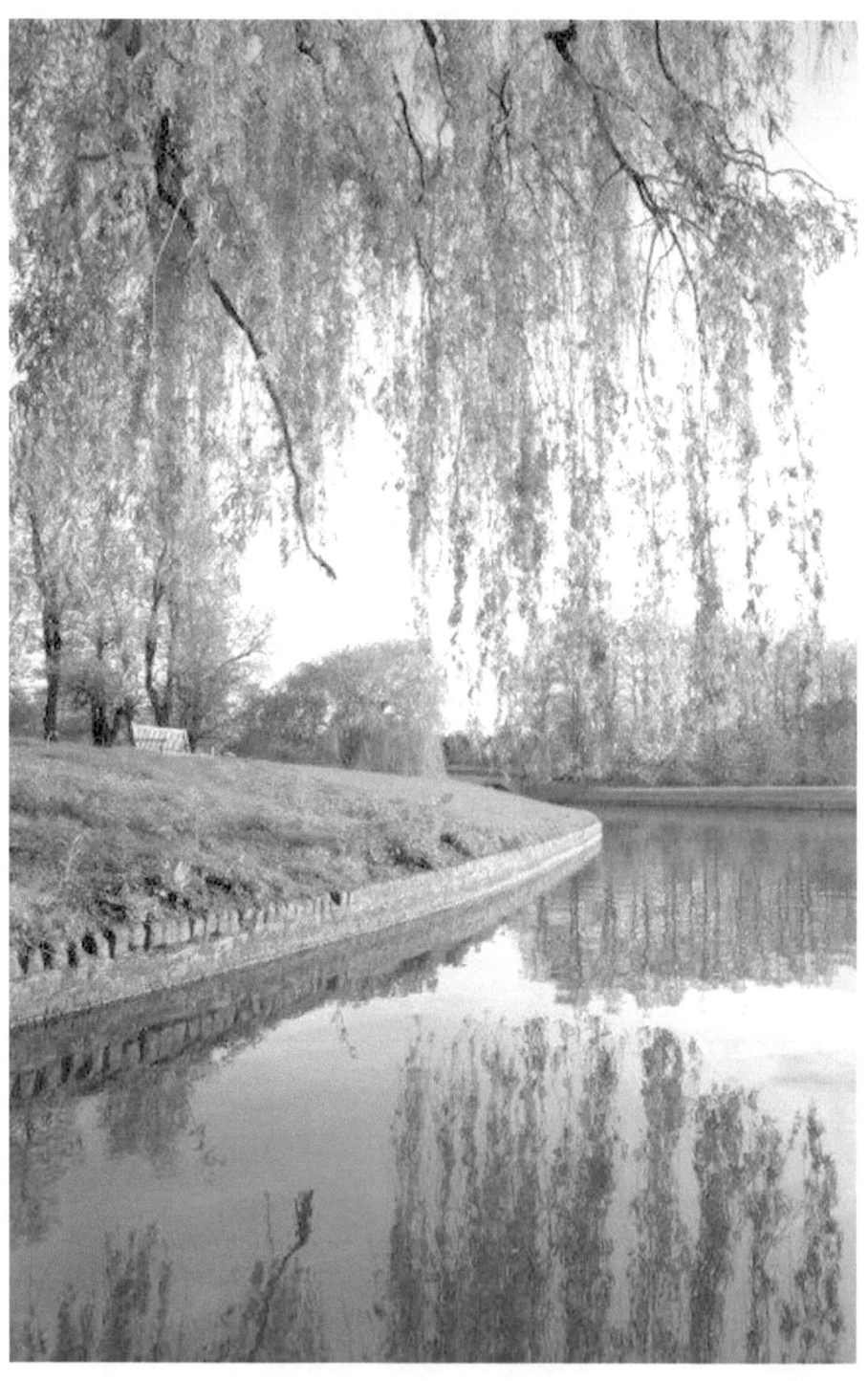

ACTIVITY LOG

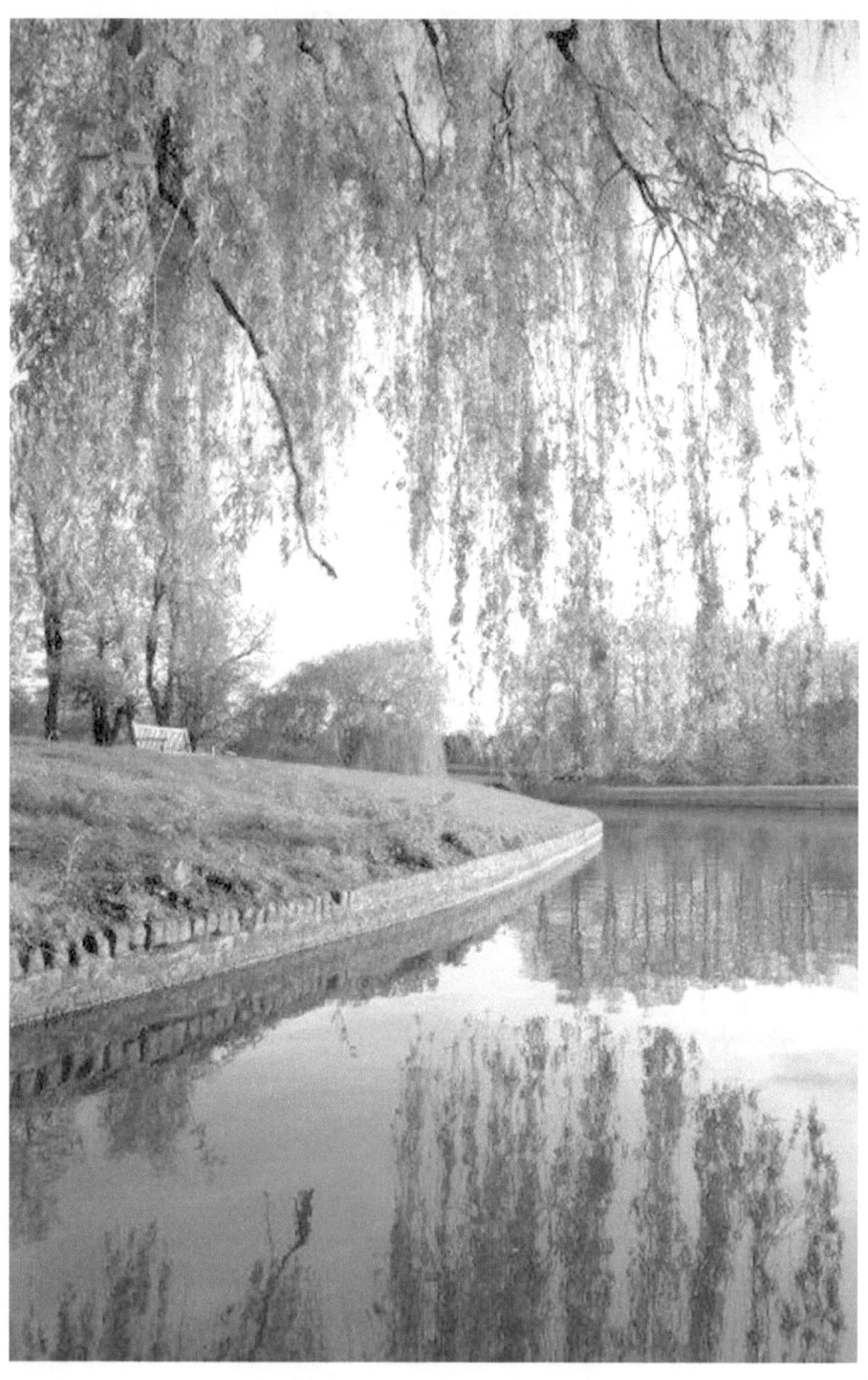

HYPERTENSION DIARY AND LOG

ACTIVITY LOG

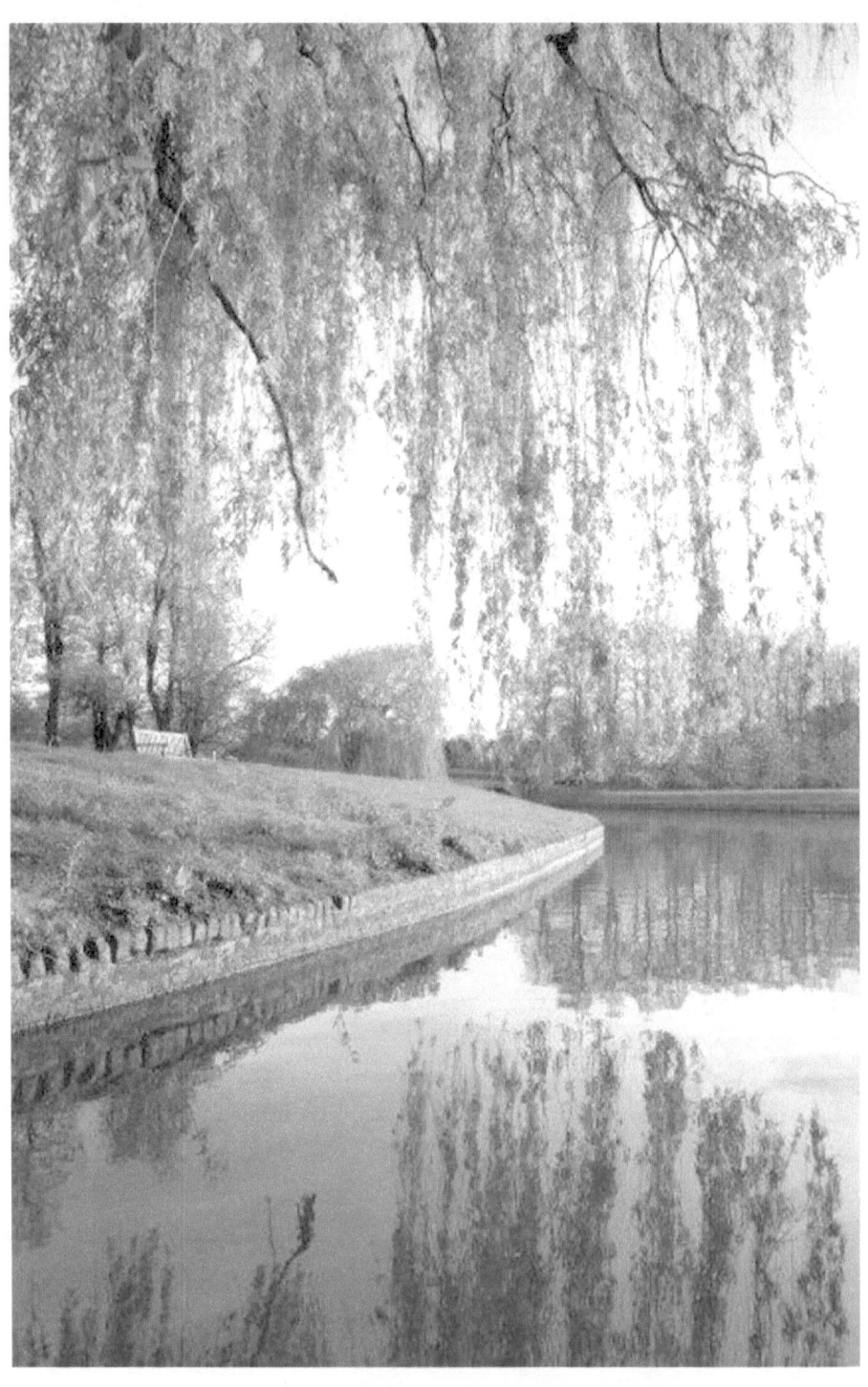

HYPERTENSION DIARY AND LOG

ACTIVITY LOG

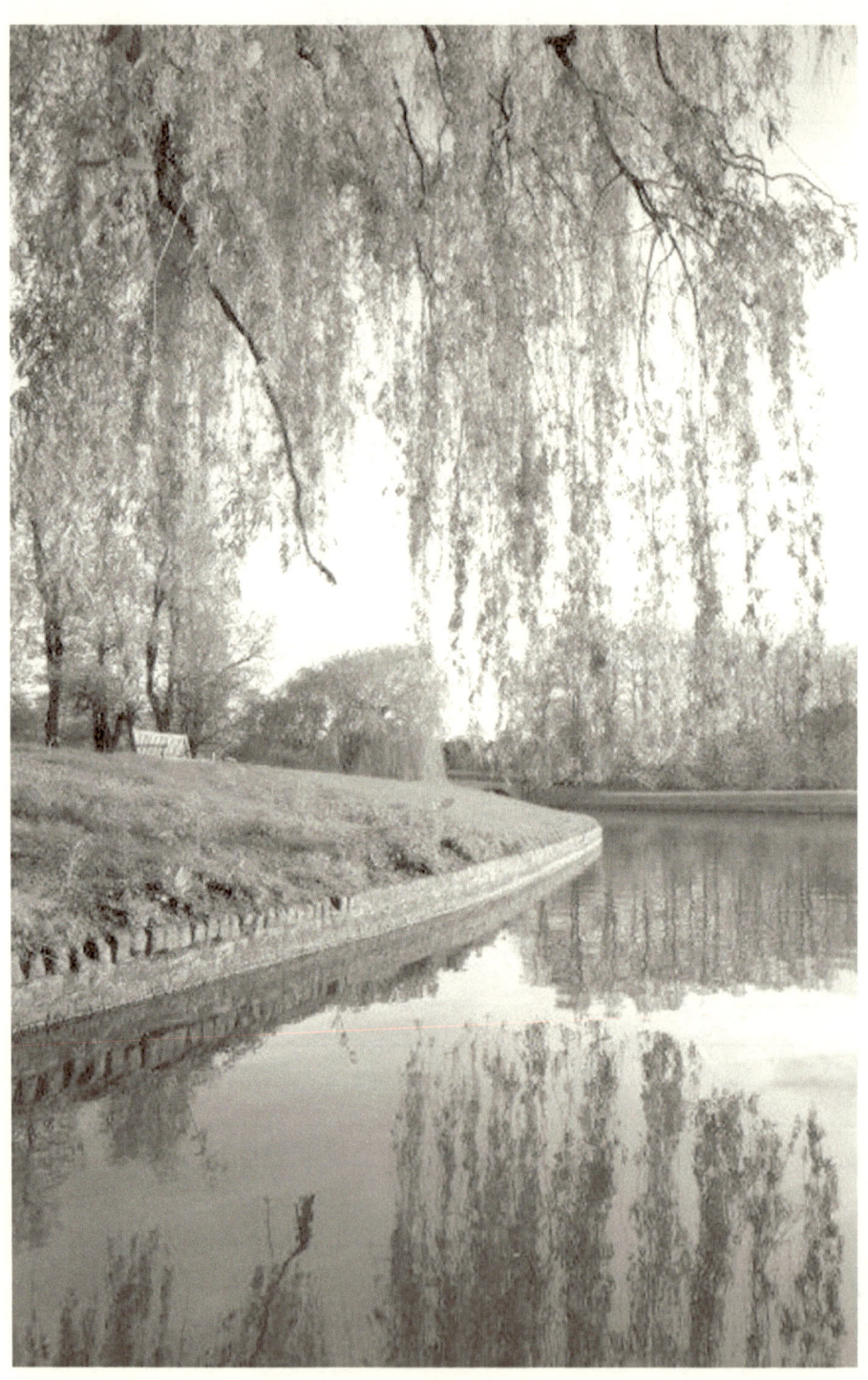

HYPERTENSION DIARY AND LOG

ACTIVITY LOG

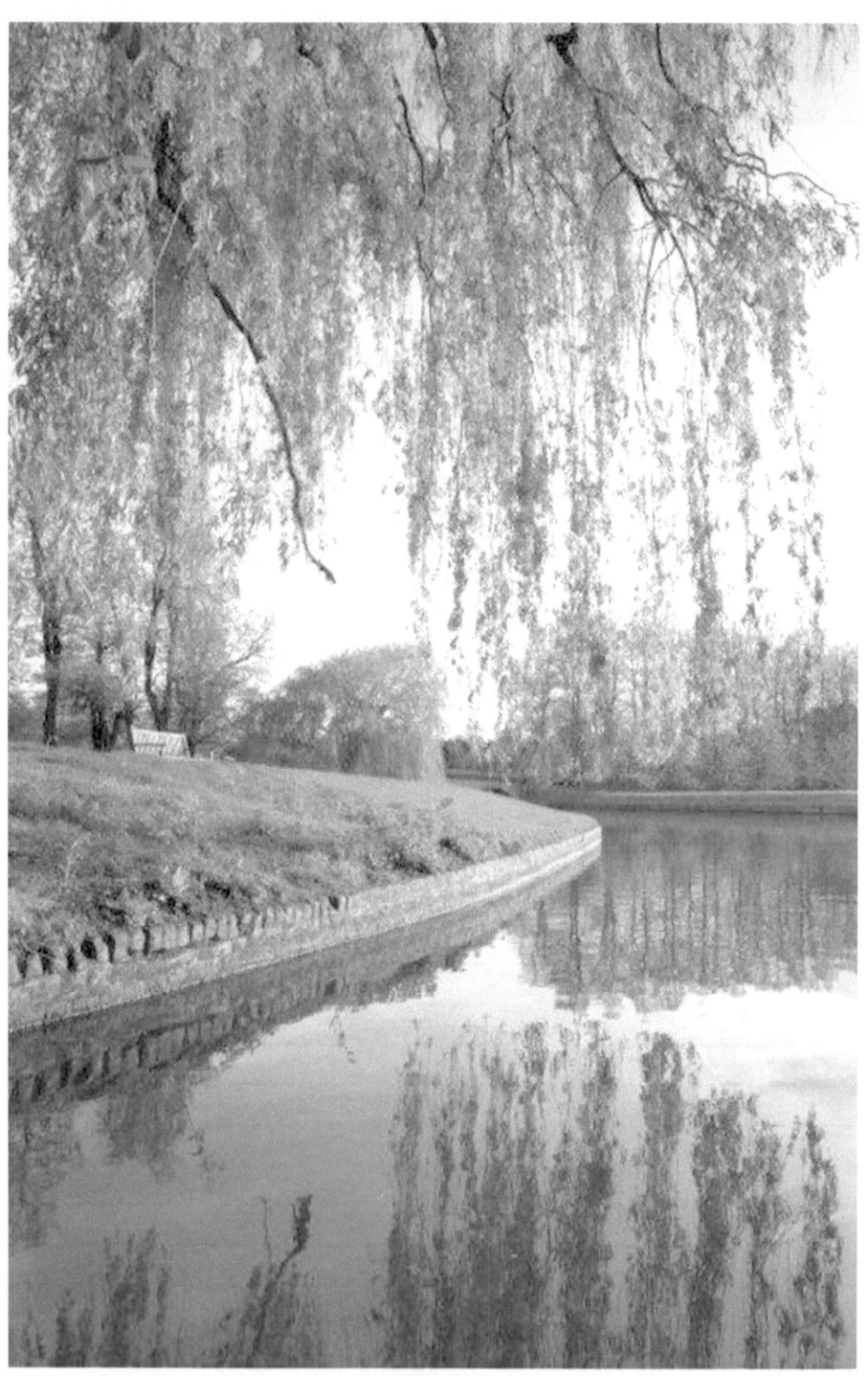

HYPERTENSION DIARY AND LOG

ACTIVITY LOG

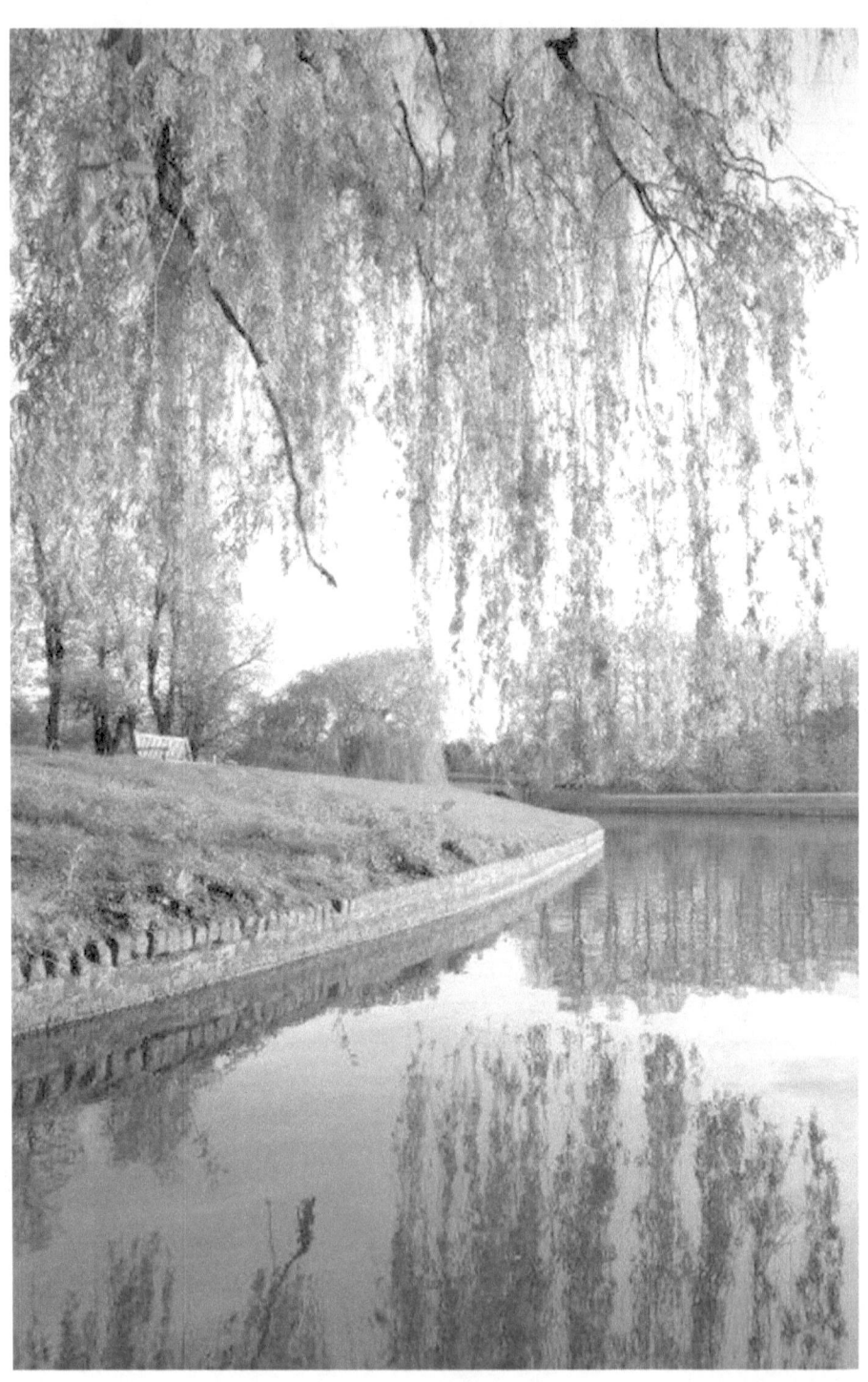

HYPERTENSION DIARY AND LOG

ACTIVITY LOG

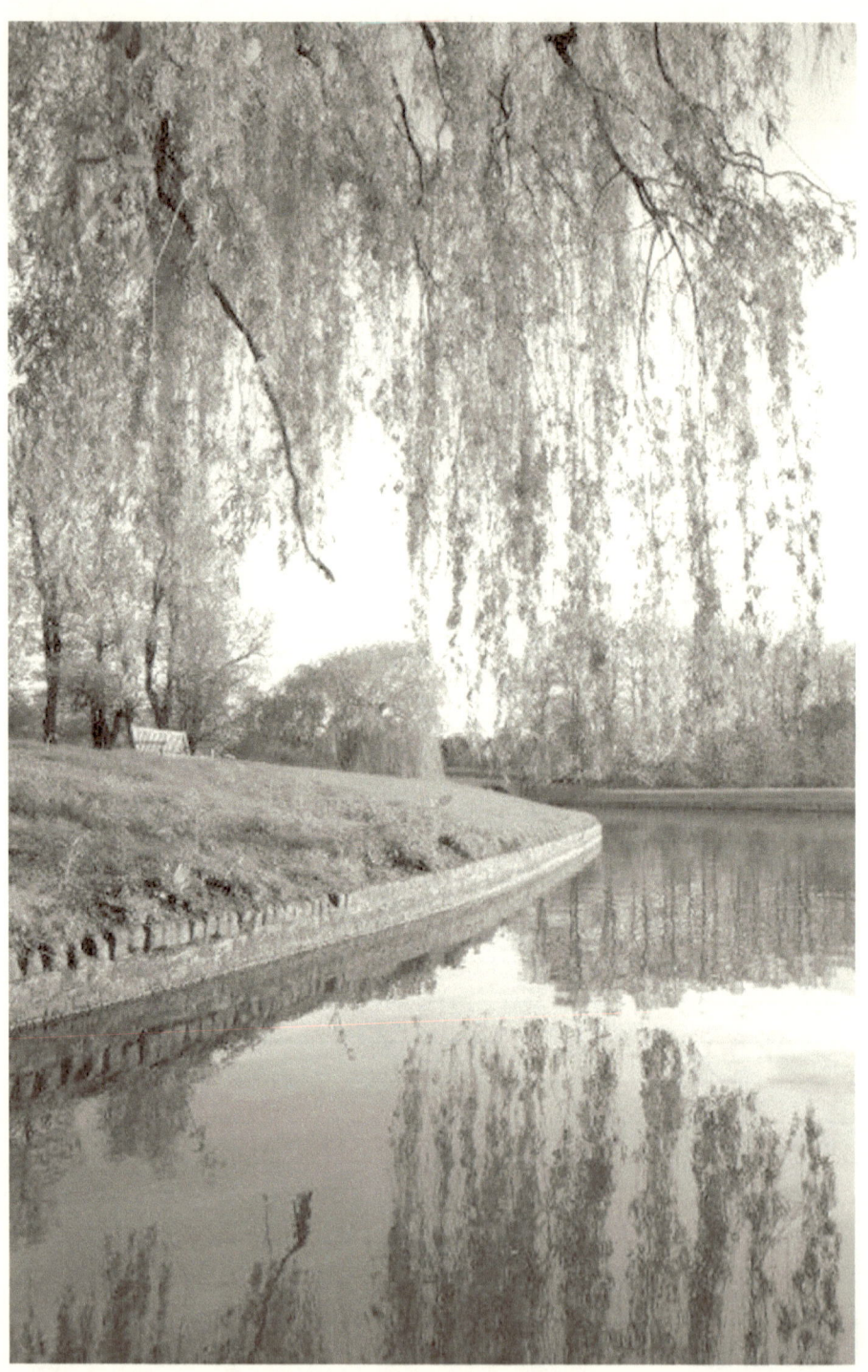

HYPERTENSION DIARY AND LOG

ACTIVITY LOG

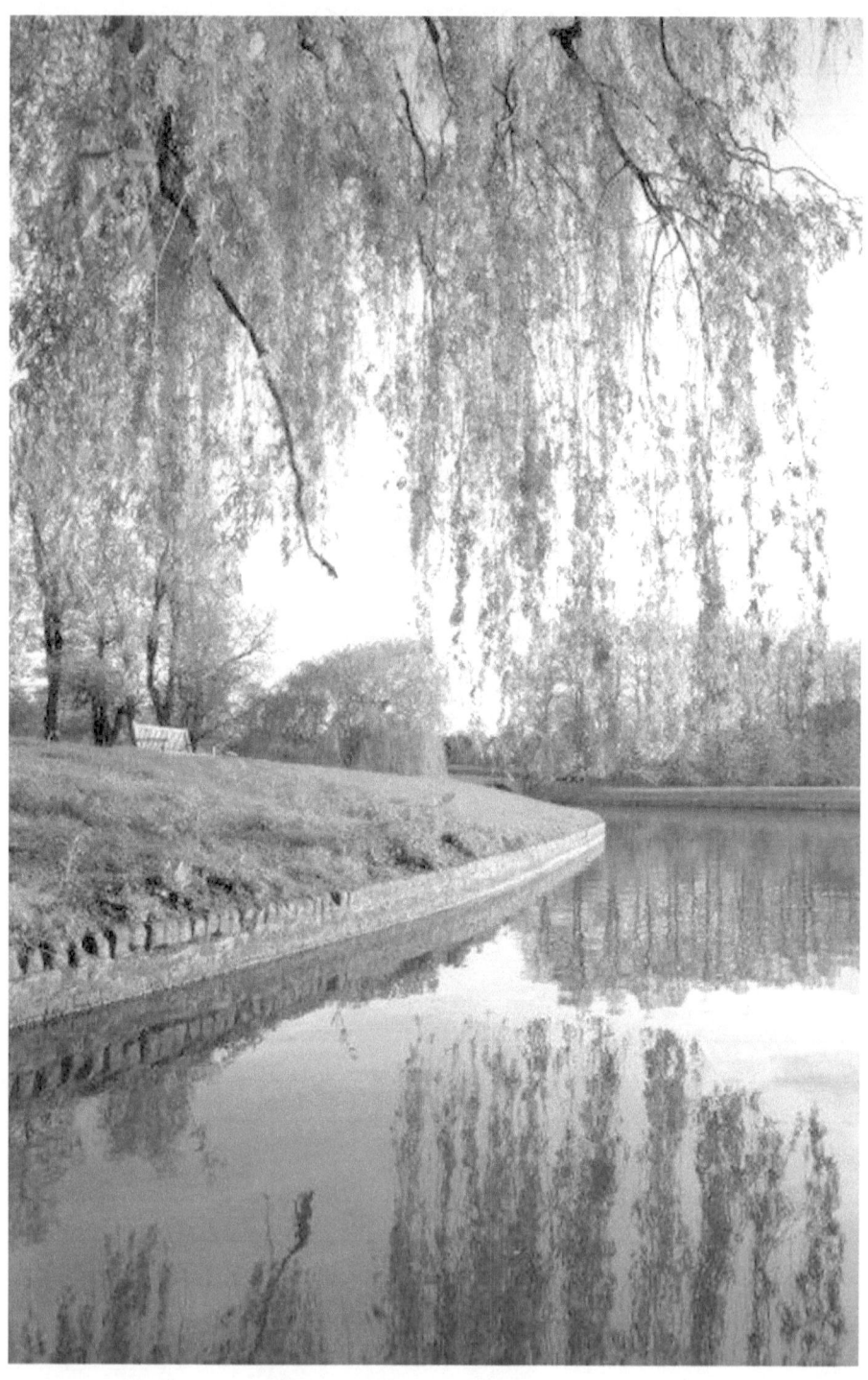

HYPERTENSION DIARY AND LOG

ACTIVITY LOG

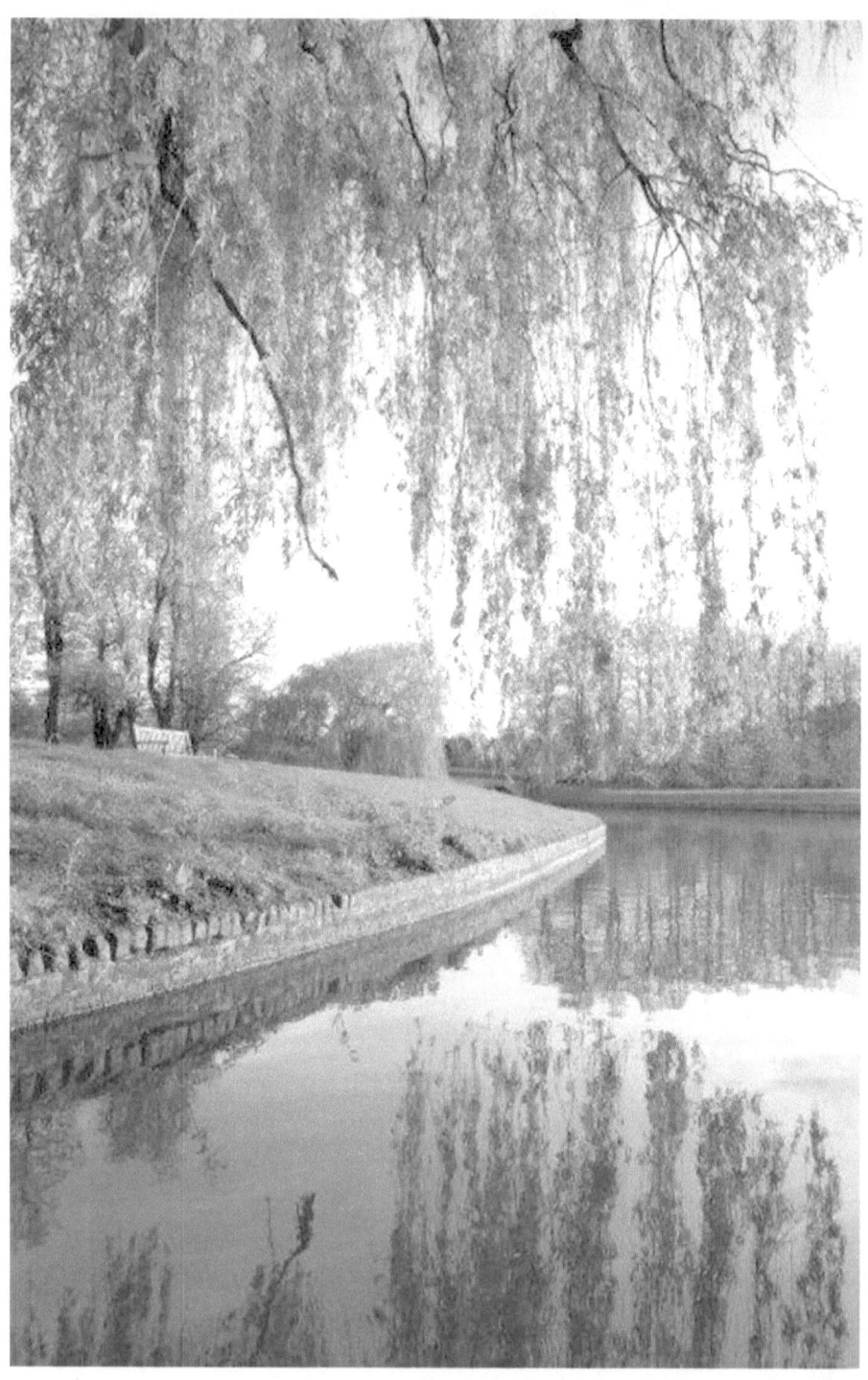

NOTES / QUESTIONS FOR DOCTOR

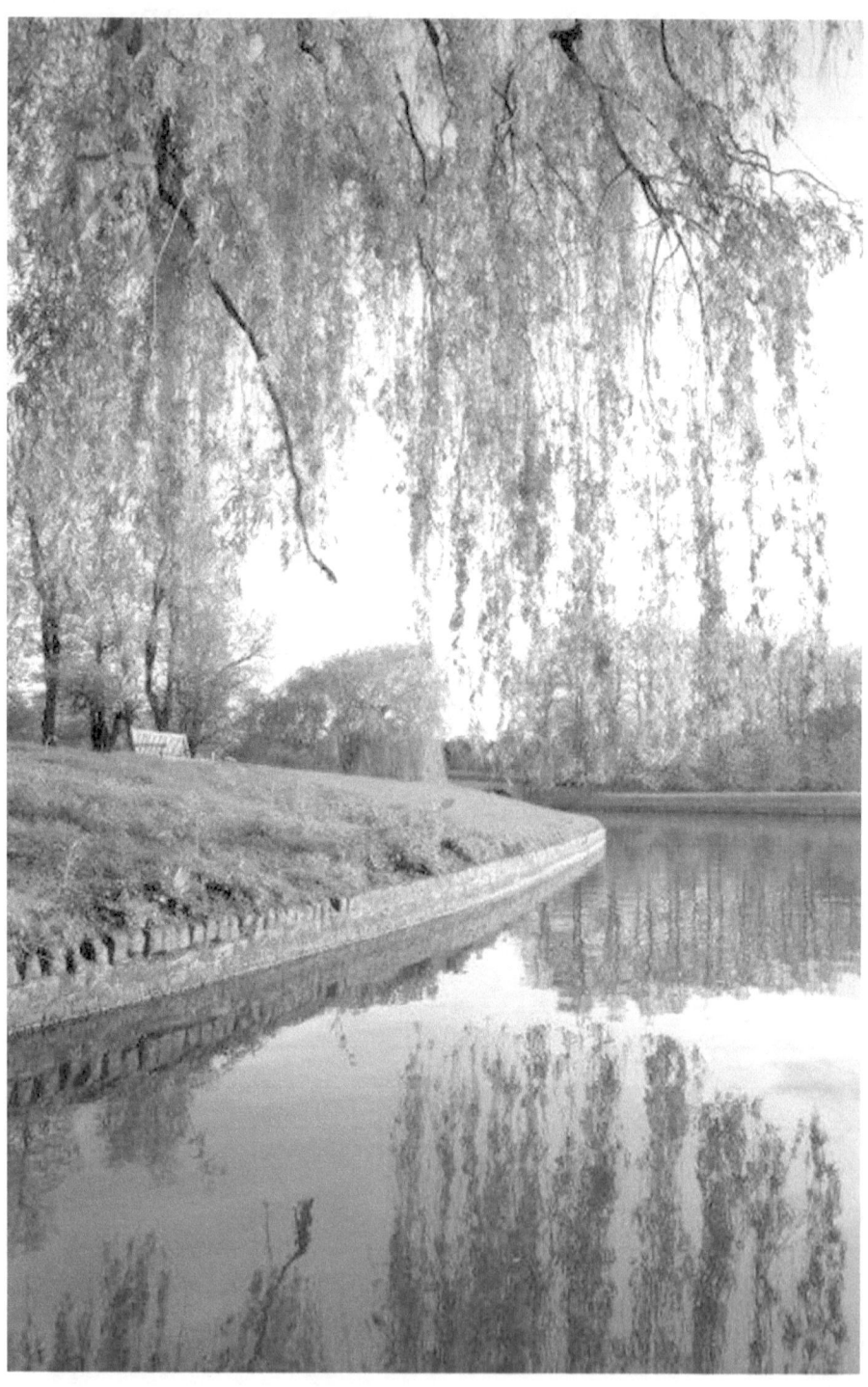

HYPERTENSION DIARY AND LOG

NOTES / QUESTIONS FOR DOCTOR

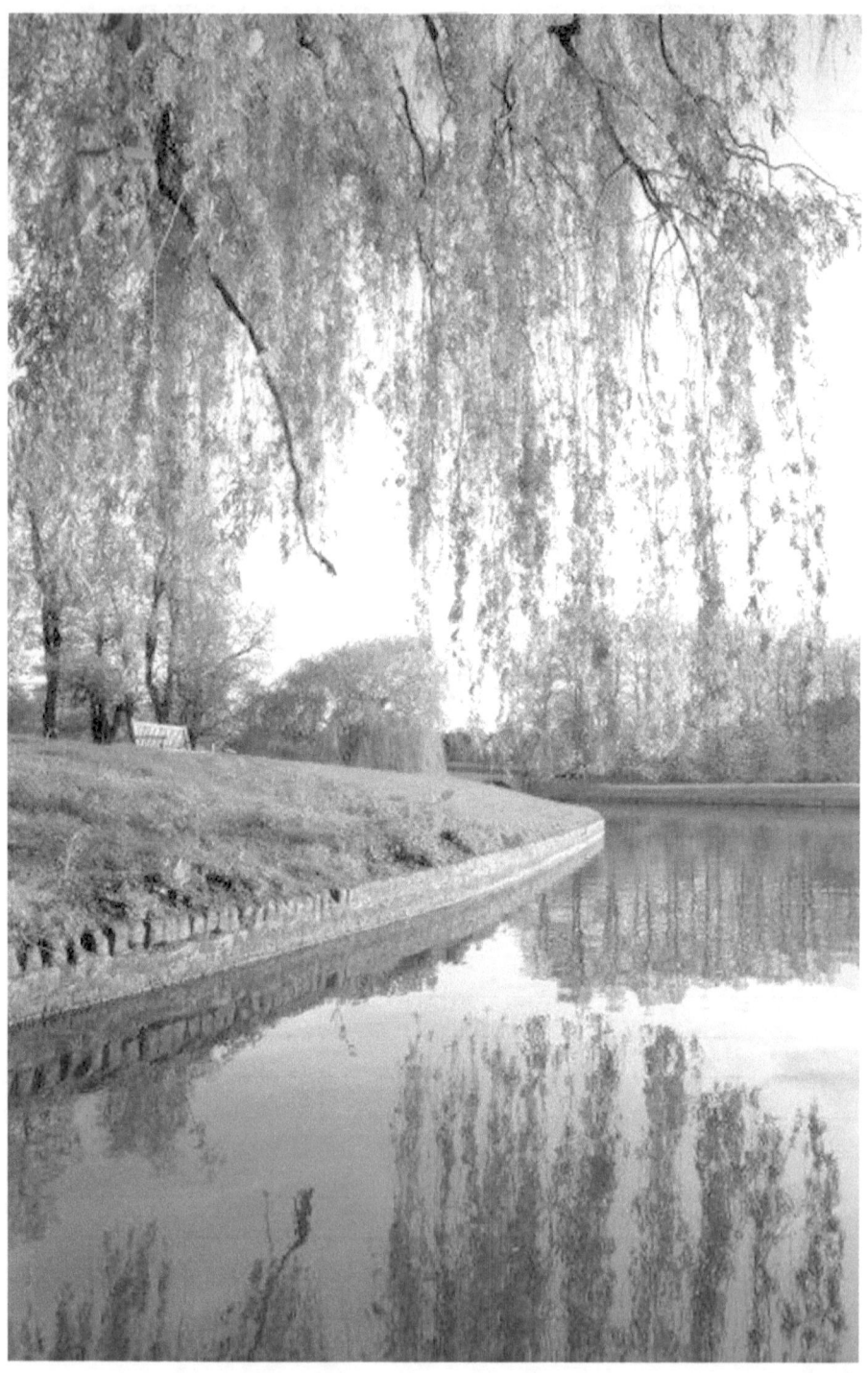

HYPERTENSION DIARY AND LOG

NOTES / QUESTIONS FOR DOCTOR

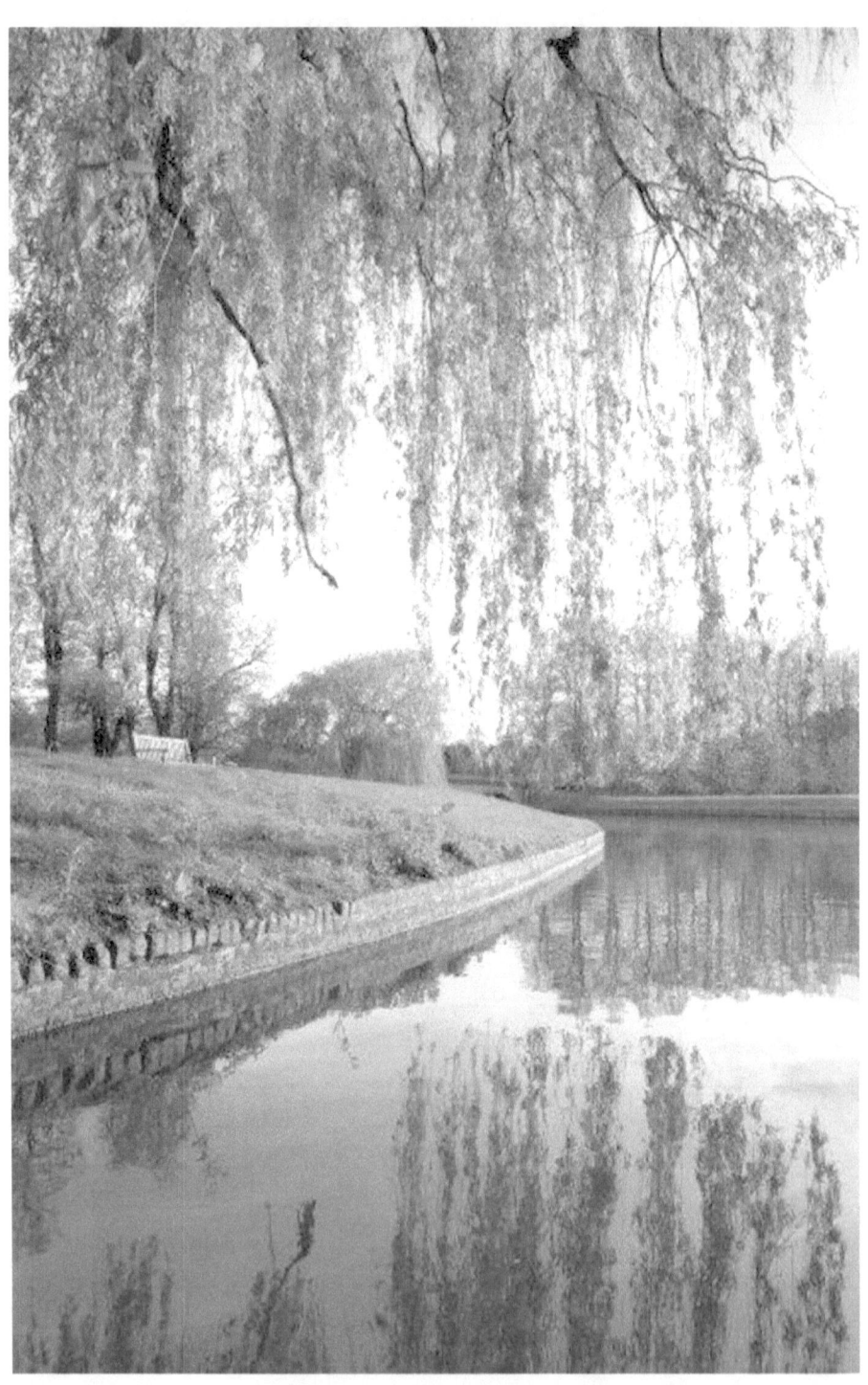

NOTES / QUESTIONS FOR DOCTOR

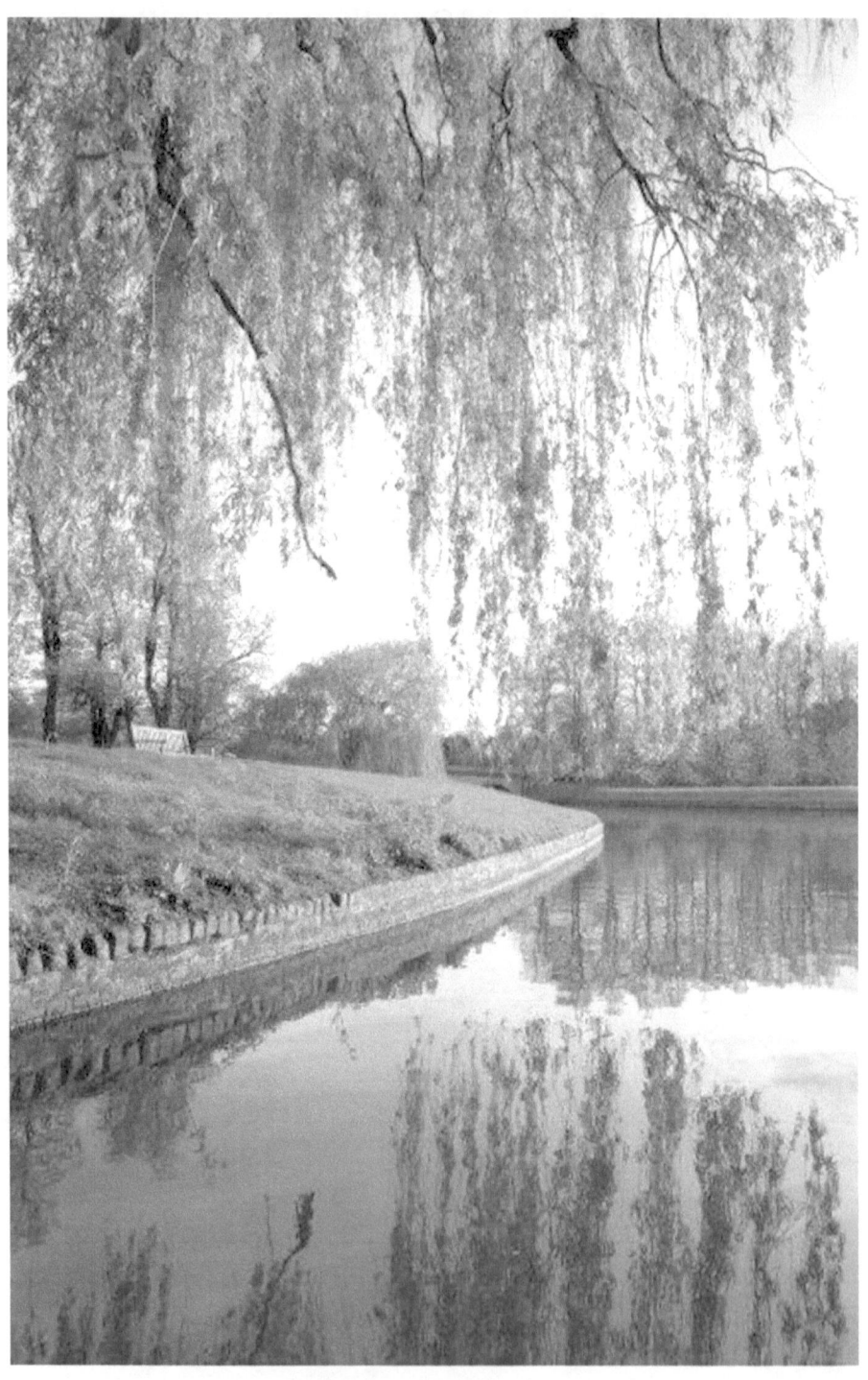

HYPERTENSION DIARY AND LOG

NOTES / QUESTIONS FOR DOCTOR

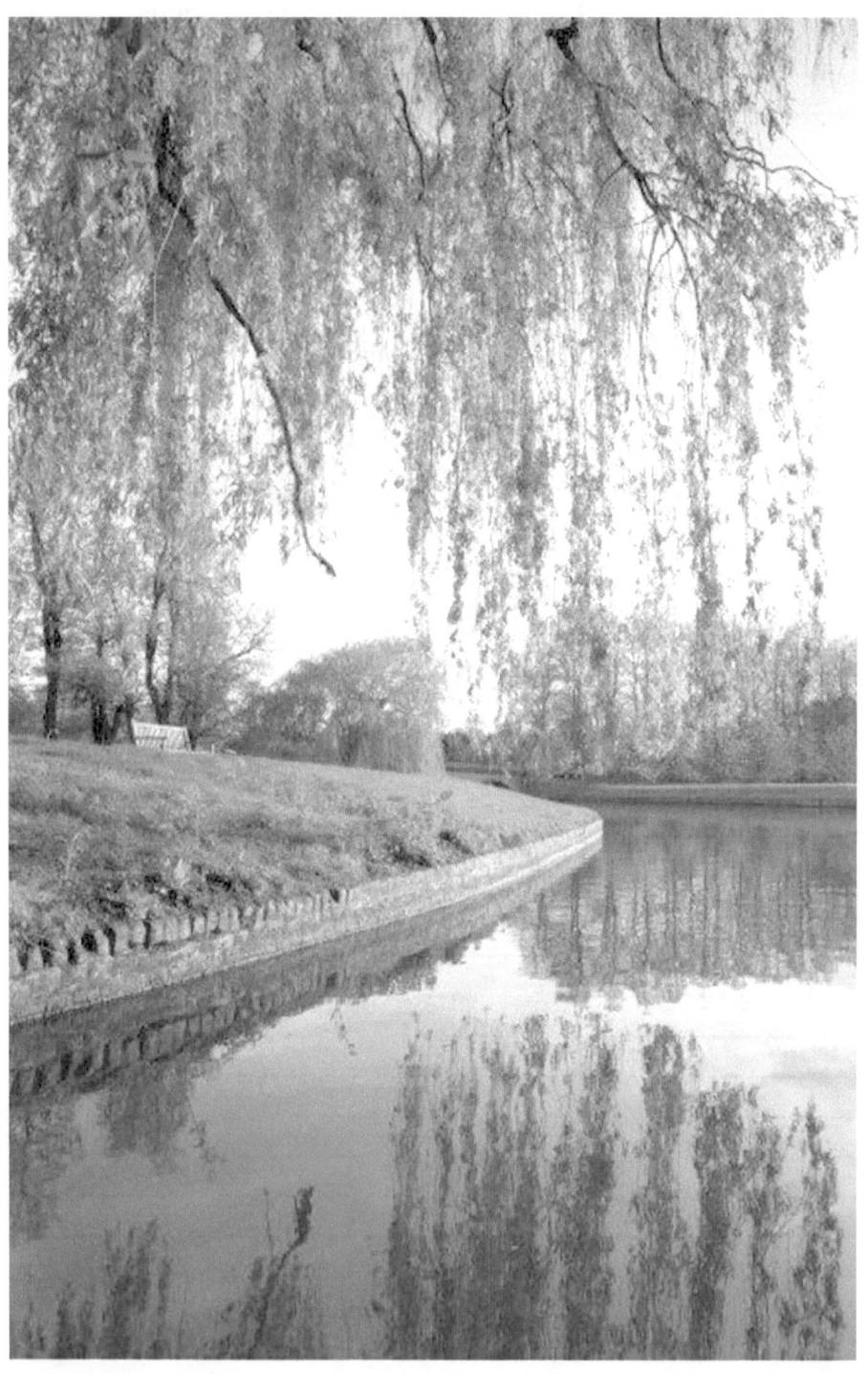

NOTES / QUESTIONS FOR DOCTOR

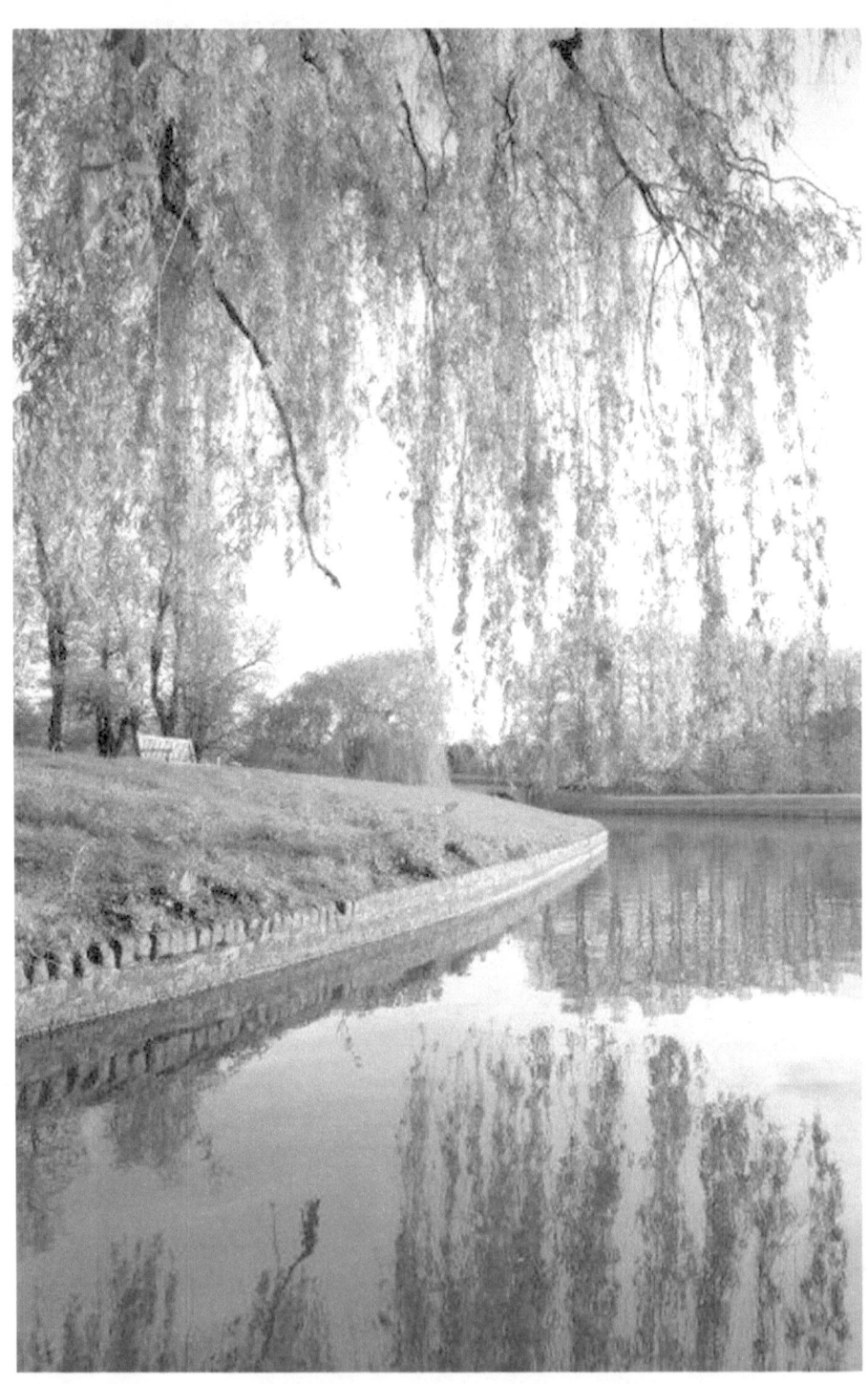

NOTES / QUESTIONS FOR DOCTOR

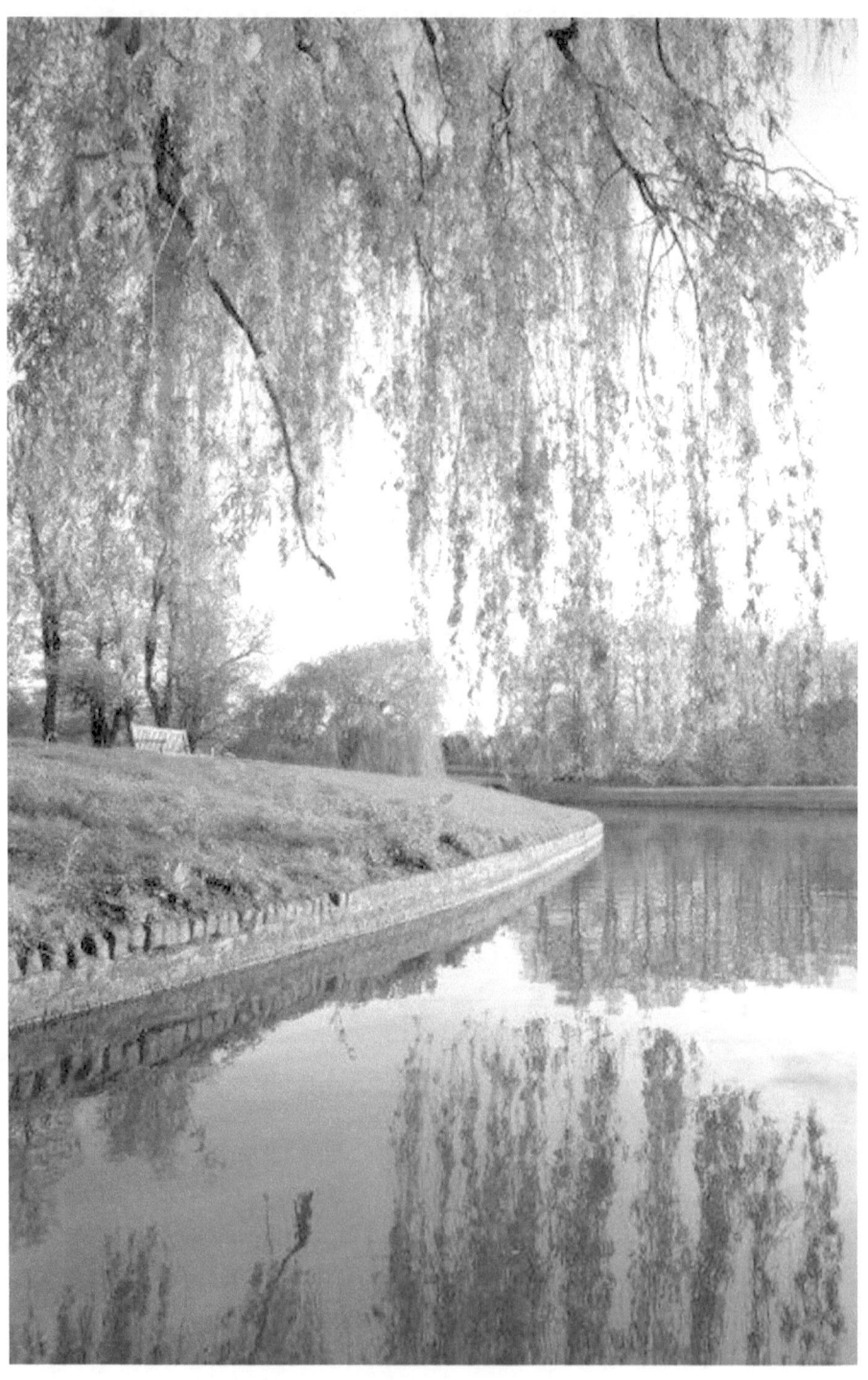

HYPERTENSION DIARY AND LOG

NOTES / QUESTIONS FOR DOCTOR

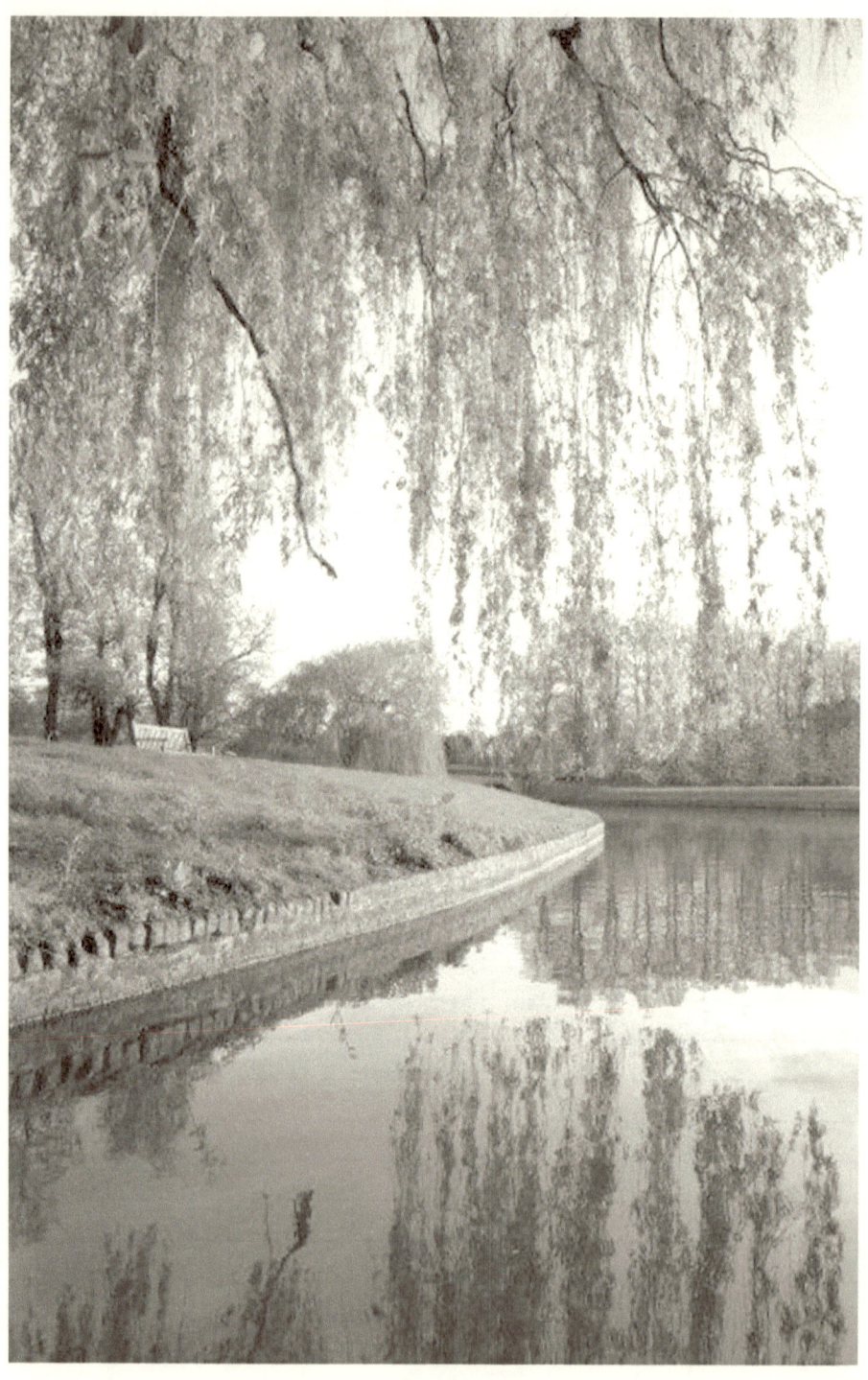

HYPERTENSION DIARY AND LOG

NOTES / QUESTIONS FOR DOCTOR

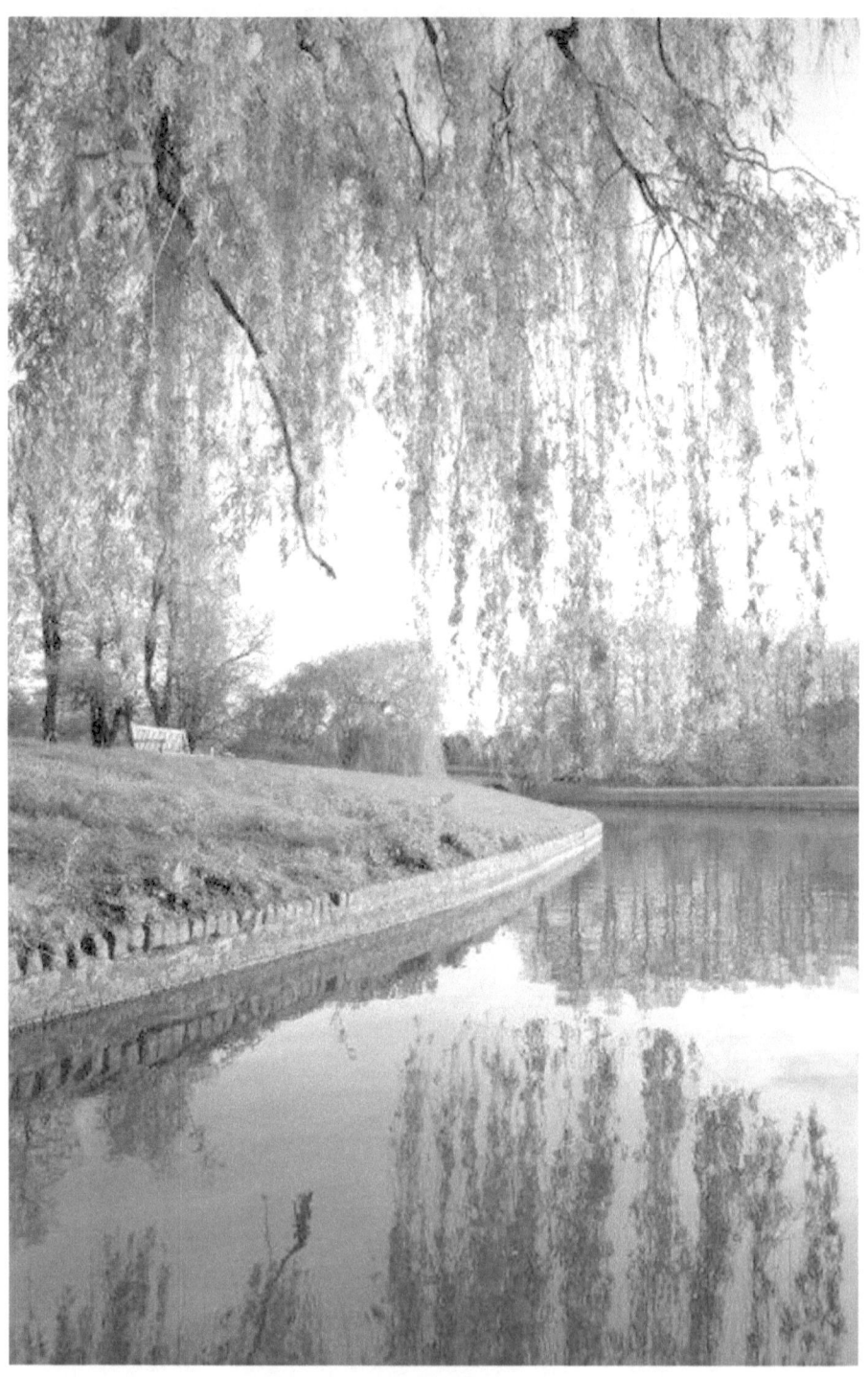

HYPERTENSION DIARY AND LOG

NOTES / QUESTIONS FOR DOCTOR

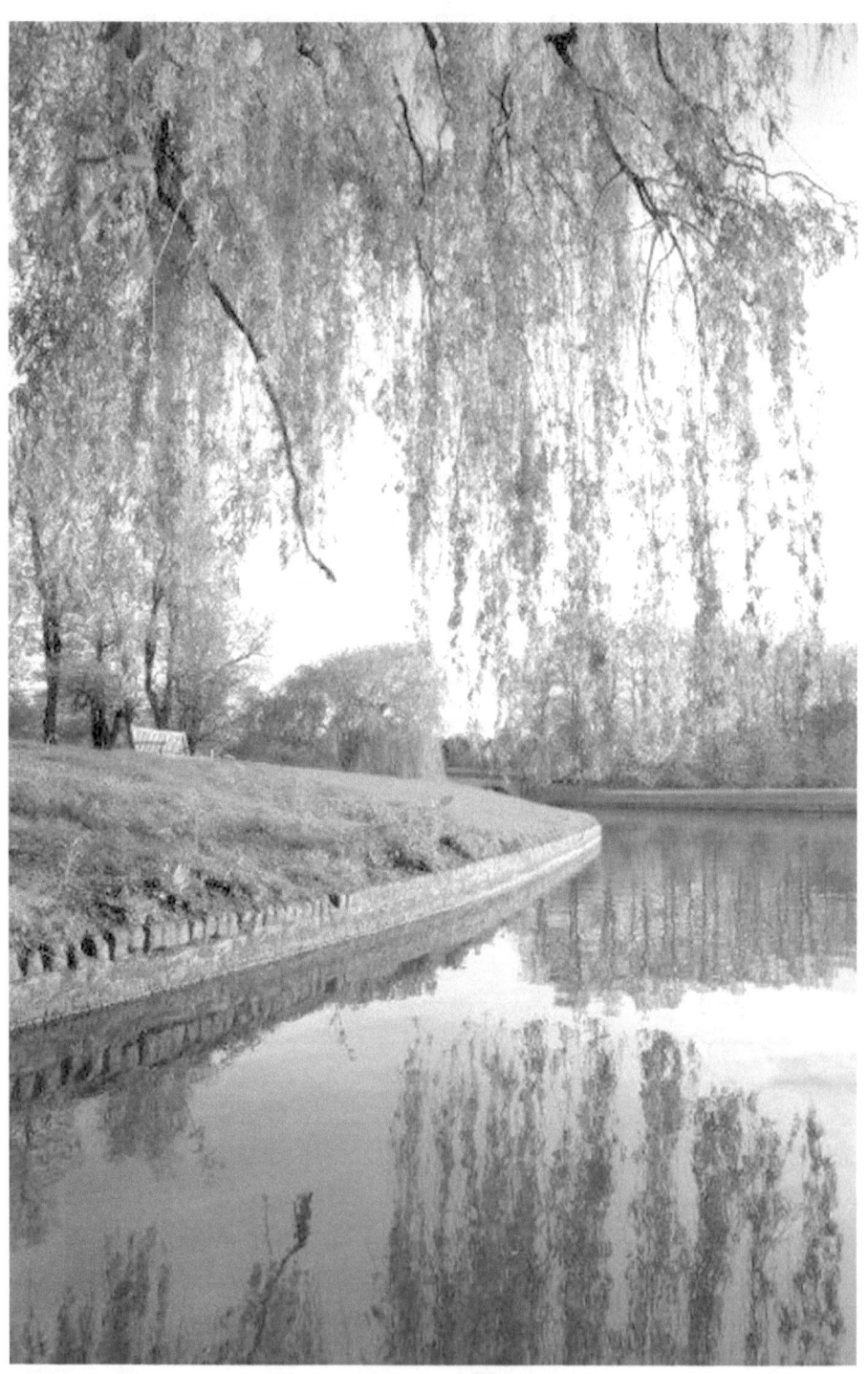

HYPERTENSION DIARY AND LOG

NOTES / QUESTIONS FOR DOCTOR

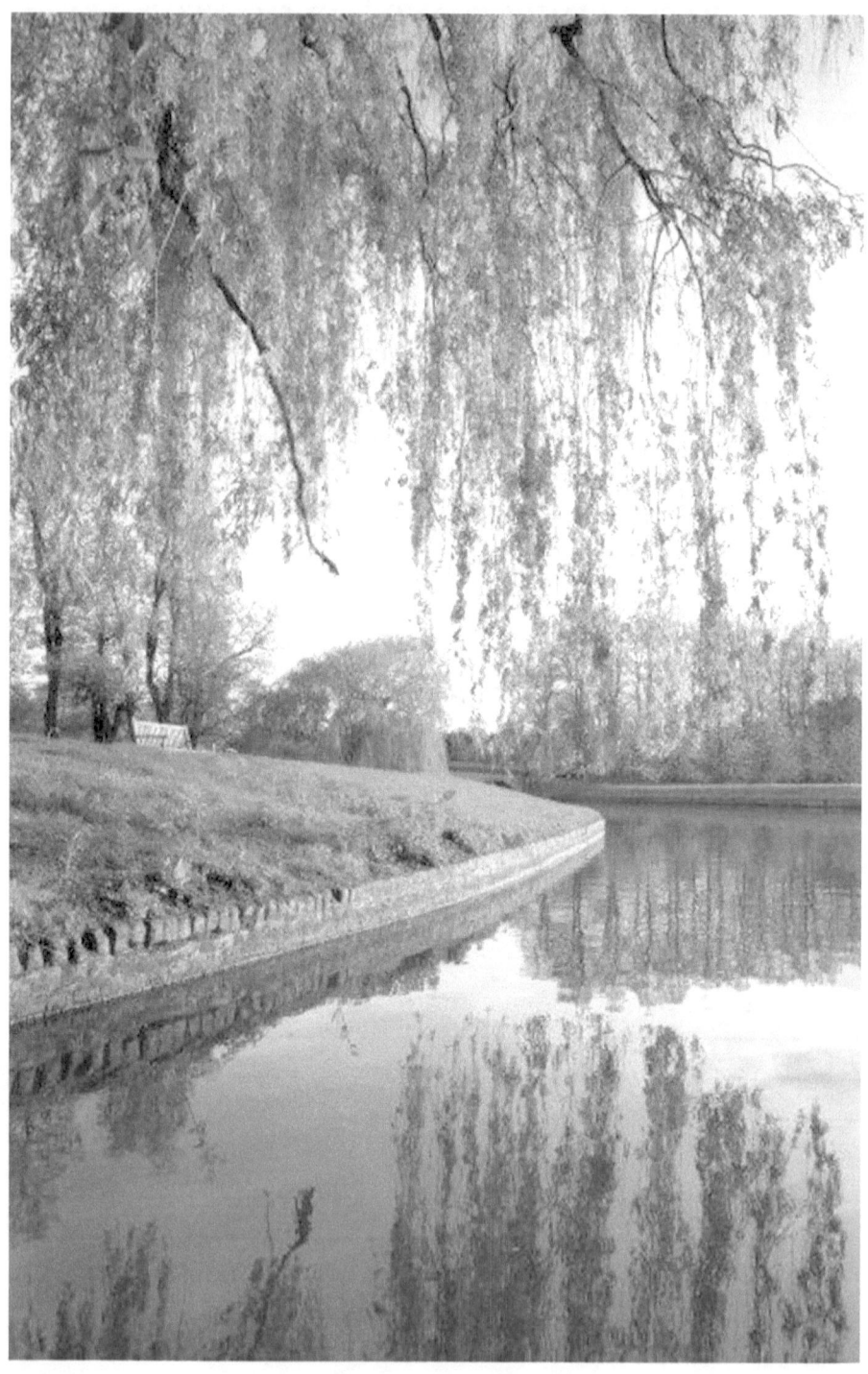

HYPERTENSION DIARY AND LOG

NOTES / QUESTIONS FOR DOCTOR

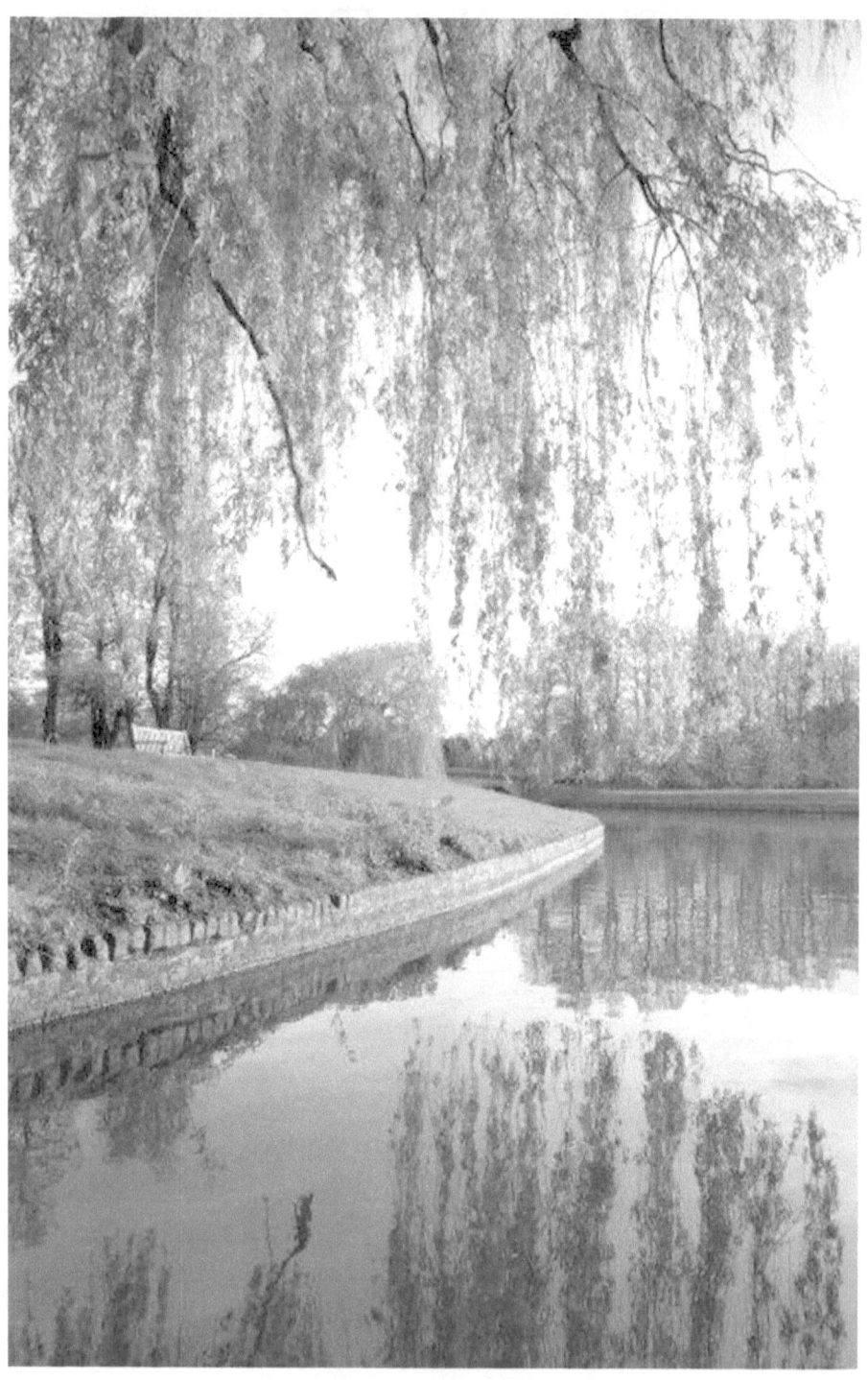

HYPERTENSION DIARY AND LOG

NOTES / QUESTIONS FOR DOCTOR

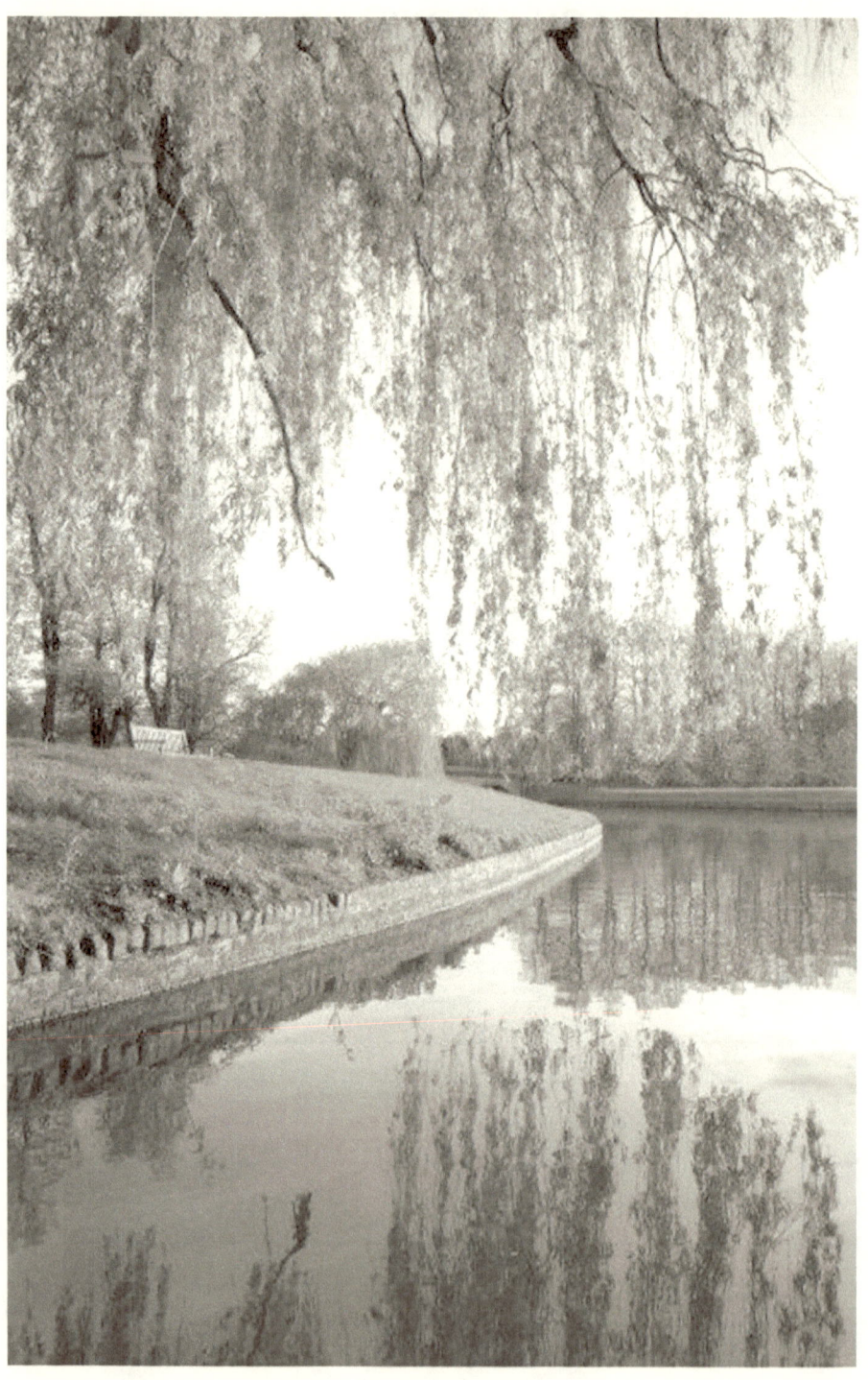

HYPERTENSION DIARY AND LOG

NOTES / QUESTIONS FOR DOCTOR

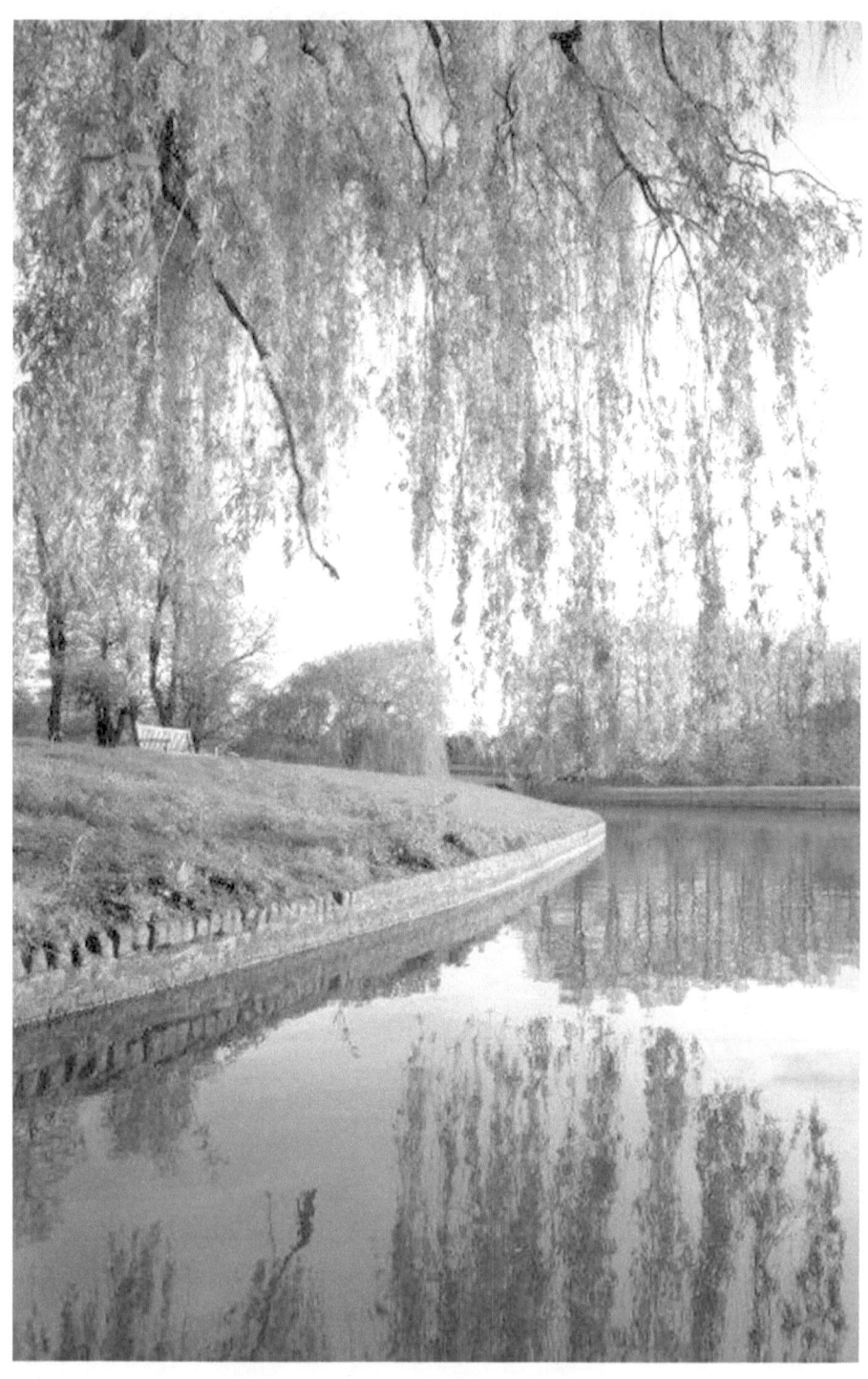

HYPERTENSION DIARY AND LOG

NOTES / QUESTIONS FOR DOCTOR

January 2011

SUNDAY	MONDAY	TUESDAY	WEDNESDAY	THURSDAY	FRIDAY	SATURDAY
						1
2	3	4	5	6	7	8
9	10	11	12	13	14	15
16	17	18	19	20	21	22
23	24	25	26	27	28	29
30	31					

HYPERTENSION DIARY AND LOG

February 2011

SUNDAY	MONDAY	TUESDAY	WEDNESDAY	THURSDAY	FRIDAY	SATURDAY
		1	2	3	4	5
6	7	8	9	10	11	12
13	14	15	16	17	18	19
20	21	22	23	24	25	26
27	28					

March 2011

SUNDAY	MONDAY	TUESDAY	WEDNESDAY	THURSDAY	FRIDAY	SATURDAY
		1	2	3	4	5
6	7	8	9	10	11	12
13	14	15	16	17	18	19
20	21	22	23	24	25	26
27	28	29	30	31		

April 2011

SUNDAY	MONDAY	TUESDAY	WEDNESDAY	THURSDAY	FRIDAY	SATURDAY
					1	2
3	4	5	6	7	8	9
10	11	12	13	14	15	16
17	18	19	20	21	22	23
24	25	26	27	28	29	30

May 2011

SUNDAY	MONDAY	TUESDAY	WEDNESDAY	THURSDAY	FRIDAY	SATURDAY
1	2	3	4	5	6	7
8	9	10	11	12	13	14
15	16	17	18	19	20	21
22	23	24	25	26	27	28
29	30	31				

June 2011

SUNDAY	MONDAY	TUESDAY	WEDNESDAY	THURSDAY	FRIDAY	SATURDAY
			1	2	3	4
5	6	7	8	9	10	11
12	13	14	15	16	17	18
19	20	21	22	23	24	25
26	27	28	29	30		

July 2011

SUNDAY	MONDAY	TUESDAY	WEDNESDAY	THURSDAY	FRIDAY	SATURDAY
					1	2
3	4	5	6	7	8	9
10	11	12	13	14	15	16
17	18	19	20	21	22	23
24	25	26	27	28	29	30
31						

HYPERTENSION DIARY AND LOG

August 2011

SUNDAY	MONDAY	TUESDAY	WEDNESDAY	THURSDAY	FRIDAY	SATURDAY
	1	2	3	4	5	6
7	8	9	10	11	12	13
14	15	16	17	18	19	20
21	22	23	24	25	26	27
28	29	30	31			

September 2011

SUNDAY	MONDAY	TUESDAY	WEDNESDAY	THURSDAY	FRIDAY	SATURDAY
				1	2	3
4	5	6	7	8	9	10
11	12	13	14	15	16	17
18	19	20	21	22	23	24
25	26	27	28	29	30	

HYPERTENSION DIARY AND LOG

October 2011

SUNDAY	MONDAY	TUESDAY	WEDNESDAY	THURSDAY	FRIDAY	SATURDAY
						1
2	3	4	5	6	7	8
9	10	11	12	13	14	15
16	17	18	19	20	21	22
23	24	25	26	27	28	29
30	31					

November 2011

SUNDAY	MONDAY	TUESDAY	WEDNESDAY	THURSDAY	FRIDAY	SATURDAY
		1	2	3	4	5
6	7	8	9	10	11	12
13	14	15	16	17	18	19
20	21	22	23	24	25	26
27	28	29	30			

HYPERTENSION DIARY AND LOG

December 2011

SUNDAY	MONDAY	TUESDAY	WEDNESDAY	THURSDAY	FRIDAY	SATURDAY
				1	2	3
4	5	6	7	8	9	10
11	12	13	14	15	16	17
18	19	20	21	22	23	24
25	26	27	28	29	30	31

January 2012

SUNDAY	MONDAY	TUESDAY	WEDNESDAY	THURSDAY	FRIDAY	SATURDAY
1	2	3	4	5	6	7
8	9	10	11	12	13	14
15	16	17	18	19	20	21
22	23	24	25	26	27	28
29	30	31				

HYPERTENSION DIARY AND LOG

February 2012

SUNDAY	MONDAY	TUESDAY	WEDNESDAY	THURSDAY	FRIDAY	SATURDAY
			1	2	3	4
5	6	7	8	9	10	11
12	13	14	15	16	17	18
19	20	21	22	23	24	25
26	27	28	29			

March 2012

SUNDAY	MONDAY	TUESDAY	WEDNESDAY	THURSDAY	FRIDAY	SATURDAY
				1	2	3
4	5	6	7	8	9	10
11	12	13	14	15	16	17
18	19	20	21	22	23	24
25	26	27	28	29	30	31

HYPERTENSION DIARY AND LOG

April 2012

SUNDAY	MONDAY	TUESDAY	WEDNESDAY	THURSDAY	FRIDAY	SATURDAY
1	2	3	4	5	6	7
8	9	10	11	12	13	14
15	16	17	18	19	20	21
22	23	24	25	26	27	28
29	30					

May 2012

SUNDAY	MONDAY	TUESDAY	WEDNESDAY	THURSDAY	FRIDAY	SATURDAY
		1	2	3	4	5
6	7	8	9	10	11	12
13	14	15	16	17	18	19
20	21	22	23	24	25	26
27	28	29	30	31		

HYPERTENSION DIARY AND LOG

June 2012

SUNDAY	MONDAY	TUESDAY	WEDNESDAY	THURSDAY	FRIDAY	SATURDAY
					1	2
3	4	5	6	7	8	9
10	11	12	13	14	15	16
17	18	19	20	21	22	23
24	25	26	27	28	29	30

July 2012

SUNDAY	MONDAY	TUESDAY	WEDNESDAY	THURSDAY	FRIDAY	SATURDAY
1	2	3	4	5	6	7
8	9	10	11	12	13	14
15	16	17	18	19	20	21
22	23	24	25	26	27	28
29	30	31				

HYPERTENSION DIARY AND LOG

August 2012

SUNDAY	MONDAY	TUESDAY	WEDNESDAY	THURSDAY	FRIDAY	SATURDAY
			1	2	3	4
5	6	7	8	9	10	11
12	13	14	15	16	17	18
19	20	21	22	23	24	25
26	27	28	29	30	31	

September 2012

SUNDAY	MONDAY	TUESDAY	WEDNESDAY	THURSDAY	FRIDAY	SATURDAY
						1
2	3	4	5	6	7	8
9	10	11	12	13	14	15
16	17	18	19	20	21	22
23	24	25	26	27	28	29
30						

October 2012

SUNDAY	MONDAY	TUESDAY	WEDNESDAY	THURSDAY	FRIDAY	SATURDAY
	1	2	3	4	5	6
7	8	9	10	11	12	13
14	15	16	17	18	19	20
21	22	23	24	25	26	27
28	29	30	31			

November 2012

SUNDAY	MONDAY	TUESDAY	WEDNESDAY	THURSDAY	FRIDAY	SATURDAY
				1	2	3
4	5	6	7	8	9	10
11	12	13	14	15	16	17
18	19	20	21	22	23	24
25	26	27	28	29	30	

December 2012

SUNDAY	MONDAY	TUESDAY	WEDNESDAY	THURSDAY	FRIDAY	SATURDAY
						1
2	3	4	5	6	7	8
9	10	11	12	13	14	15
16	17	18	19	20	21	22
23	24	25	26	27	28	29
30	31					

January 2013

SUNDAY	MONDAY	TUESDAY	WEDNESDAY	THURSDAY	FRIDAY	SATURDAY
		1	2	3	4	5
6	7	8	9	10	11	12
13	14	15	16	17	18	19
20	21	22	23	24	25	26
27	28	29	30	31		

HYPERTENSION DIARY AND LOG

February 2013

SUNDAY	MONDAY	TUESDAY	WEDNESDAY	THURSDAY	FRIDAY	SATURDAY
					1	2
3	4	5	6	7	8	9
10	11	12	13	14	15	16
17	18	19	20	21	22	23
24	25	26	27	28		

March 2013

SUNDAY	MONDAY	TUESDAY	WEDNESDAY	THURSDAY	FRIDAY	SATURDAY
					1	2
3	4	5	6	7	8	9
10	11	12	13	14	15	16
17	18	19	20	21	22	23
24	25	26	27	28	29	30
31						

April 2013

SUNDAY	MONDAY	TUESDAY	WEDNESDAY	THURSDAY	FRIDAY	SATURDAY
	1	2	3	4	5	6
7	8	9	10	11	12	13
14	15	16	17	18	19	20
21	22	23	24	25	26	27
28	29	30				

May 2013

SUNDAY	MONDAY	TUESDAY	WEDNESDAY	THURSDAY	FRIDAY	SATURDAY
			1	2	3	4
5	6	7	8	9	10	11
12	13	14	15	16	17	18
19	20	21	22	23	24	25
26	27	28	29	30	31	

June 2013

SUNDAY	MONDAY	TUESDAY	WEDNESDAY	THURSDAY	FRIDAY	SATURDAY
						1
2	3	4	5	6	7	8
9	10	11	12	13	14	15
16	17	18	19	20	21	22
23	24	25	26	27	28	29
30						

July 2013

SUNDAY	MONDAY	TUESDAY	WEDNESDAY	THURSDAY	FRIDAY	SATURDAY
	1	2	3	4	5	6
7	8	9	10	11	12	13
14	15	16	17	18	19	20
21	22	23	24	25	26	27
28	29	30	31			

August 2013

SUNDAY	MONDAY	TUESDAY	WEDNESDAY	THURSDAY	FRIDAY	SATURDAY
				1	2	3
4	5	6	7	8	9	10
11	12	13	14	15	16	17
18	19	20	21	22	23	24
25	26	27	28	29	30	31

September 2013

SUNDAY	MONDAY	TUESDAY	WEDNESDAY	THURSDAY	FRIDAY	SATURDAY
1	2	3	4	5	6	7
8	9	10	11	12	13	14
15	16	17	18	19	20	21
22	23	24	25	26	27	28
29	30					

October 2013

SUNDAY	MONDAY	TUESDAY	WEDNESDAY	THURSDAY	FRIDAY	SATURDAY
		1	2	3	4	5
6	7	8	9	10	11	12
13	14	15	16	17	18	19
20	21	22	23	24	25	26
27	28	29	30	31		

November 2013

SUNDAY	MONDAY	TUESDAY	WEDNESDAY	THURSDAY	FRIDAY	SATURDAY
					1	2
3	4	5	6	7	8	9
10	11	12	13	14	15	16
17	18	19	20	21	22	23
24	25	26	27	28	29	30

HYPERTENSION DIARY AND LOG

December 2013

SUNDAY	MONDAY	TUESDAY	WEDNESDAY	THURSDAY	FRIDAY	SATURDAY
1	2	3	4	5	6	7
8	9	10	11	12	13	14
15	16	17	18	19	20	21
22	23	24	25	26	27	28
29	30	31